BAD MEDICINE

David Wootton is Anniversary Professor of History at the University of York. He has published widely in early modern intellectual history, particularly on the history of political thought, and is a regular reviewer for the *London Review of Books* and the *Times Literary Supplement*.

BAD MEDICINE

DOCTORS DOING HARM
SINCE HIPPOCRATES

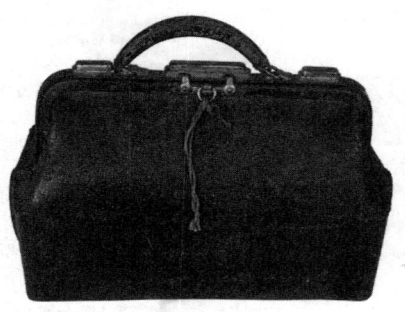

DAVID WOOTTON

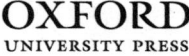

OXFORD
UNIVERSITY PRESS

OXFORD
UNIVERSITY PRESS

Great Clarendon Street, Oxford OX2 6DP

Oxford University Press is a department of the University of Oxford.
It furthers the University's objective of excellence in research, scholarship,
and education by publishing worldwide in

Oxford New York

Auckland Cape Town Dar es Salaam Hong Kong Karachi
Kuala Lumpur Madrid Melbourne Mexico City Nairobi
New Delhi Shanghai Taipei Toronto

With offices in

Argentina Austria Brazil Chile Czech Republic France Greece
Guatemala Hungary Italy Japan Poland Portugal Singapore
South Korea Switzerland Thailand Turkey Ukraine Vietnam

Oxford is a registered trade mark of Oxford University Press
in the UK and in certain other countries

Published in the United States
by Oxford University Press Inc., New York

British Library Cataloguing in Publication Data

Data available

Library of Congress Cataloging in Publication Data

Data available

Typeset by RefineCatch Limited, Bungay, Suffolk
Printed in Great Britain by
Clays Limited, St Ives plc

ISBN 978–0–19–280355–9 (Hbk.)
978–0–19–921279–8 (Pbk.)

Praise for *Bad Medicine*:

'An inspiring account of individual accomplishment'
Daily Telegraph

'A very stimulating and thought-provoking book'
Sunday Telegraph

'A fascinating story'
Sunday Times

'Ought to be required reading for every first year medical student.'
British Medical Journal

'A genuinely thrilling adventure . . . emotionally and intellectually
gripping . . . the historical catastrophe of medicine has never been so
excitingly and stirringly told.'
Times Literary Supplement

'Shockingly persuasive.'
The Scotsman

'A wonderfully iconoclastic challenge to approaches taken by other
historians.'
Sir Iain Chalmers, Editor, James Lind Library

'Anyone with an involvement with medicine—and that means
anyone with a body and a brain—should read this brilliant, bracing
and erudite book.'
Seamus Sweeney, Social Affairs Unit

'Sometimes it happens that a sober-eyed historian with a flair for
writing . . . presents us with a picture of the world that we are not
used to seeing. He invites us to think in a fresh, creative way that
allows us to learn from the past and move away from the fossilized
mentality of the medical profession.'
Haaretz

ACKNOWLEDGEMENTS

Alison Mark first suggested this project. Katharine Reeve commissioned it. Luciana O'Flaherty adopted it. Students at Queen Mary, University of London, and at the University of York explored the subject with me. The University of York gave me a sabbatical in which to write. Audiences at Birkbeck, University of London; the History of Science Seminar in the University of Cambridge; the Department of History in the University of York; and the National Humanities Centre at Ralegh-Durham discussed chapters with me. Harold Cook, Lauren Kassell, Stuart Reynolds, and Lisa Wootton read a draft, and I am grateful for their comments. They are not responsible for my errors, nor my failings. Nor, of course, is Alison Mark, who has kept company with this project from beginning to end. The paperback edition has benefited from discussions with Robin Briggs (on scurvy—which has resulted in substantial rewriting on p. 161), with Iain Chalmers (which has led to some changes in my account of the history of clinical trials), and with Michael MacKay (on William Taplin).

CONTENTS

NOTE ON SOURCES

This book is not burdened with numerous footnotes and a lengthy bibliography, though I know it will be read by students and scholars as well as by others with an interest in the subject. For those who wish to pursue this further, at www.badmedicine.co.uk you will find detailed bibliographies and notes, along with links to other web sites. You will also find updates: corrections, clarifications, responses to critics, and references to literature that has appeared since this book was written. The very short bibliography you will find at the end is intended only as an indication of the most important sources on which I have drawn and the most significant works that have influenced my thinking.

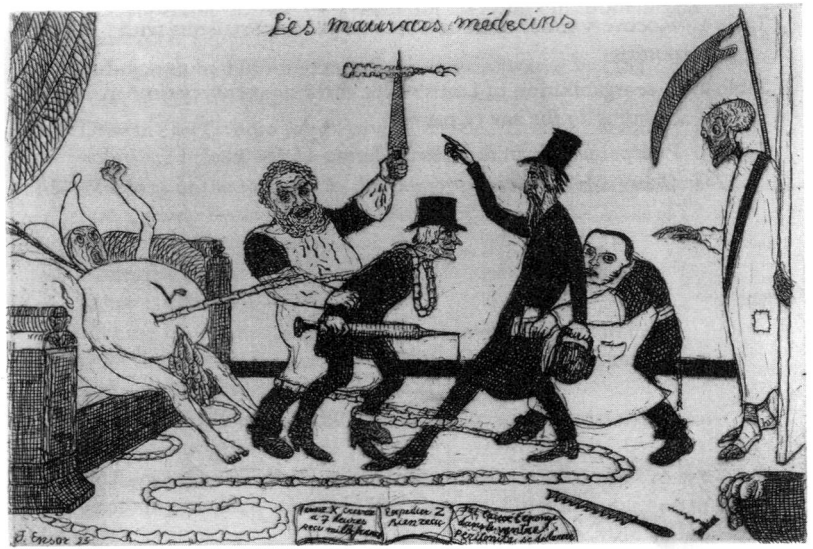

1. James Ensor, *The Bad Doctors*, 1895. Etching. Three doctors, working with crude instruments (a carpenter's saw, a corkscrew) have been performing abdominal surgery on a helpless patient – they have even removed his backbone.

INTRODUCTION: BAD MEDICINE/ BETTER MEDICINE

We all have bodies, and all our bodies function in much the same way. Each of us originates in a fertilized egg; we all breathe and maintain a heartbeat; we all eat, digest, and excrete. If we cannot perform these basic functions for ourselves, then our life depends on medical machinery doing them for us. In these respects we are all alike, and like, too, not only all the generations of human beings before us, but all mammals, birds, and reptiles. Bodies, you could say, have no history because they have been much the same since the first human beings came into existence.

But our bodies do have a history. I am tall, over six feet. The vast majority of people over six feet tall have been born in the last century, perhaps in the last thirty years. In the mid-eighteenth century Frederick the Great of Prussia searched across Europe to assemble a regiment of men over six foot tall: the enterprise took its point from the rarity of such giants. Anybody inspecting my body for a post mortem would find that on my upper arm there is the scar of a vaccination against smallpox, which must have occurred after 1796, when Jenner invented vaccination, and before 1980, when smallpox was officially declared eradicated. They would also find evidence of my surviving an appendix operation and a compound fracture of the tibia: this, as we shall see, implies medical care received after 1865. Before that date an appendectomy was almost certain to be fatal, while the only hope for someone with a compound fracture (where the bone sticks through the skin) was amputation. The amalgams used to repair my teeth, and my varifocal lenses, without which I would be half blind, set a *terminus post quem* in the late twentieth century. My life expectancy is quite different from that of someone born a hundred or a thousand years ago. Put two dead bodies, one from the eleventh century and one from any industrialized society in the twenty-first, on to a mortuary slab, and you would not need to be an expert to tell them apart.

To have a body is to experience, at least on occasion, pain: every infant suffers from wind and teething. Every child encounters disease. And part of the process of growing up is discovering that death awaits us all. All societies seek to alleviate pain, ward off disease, and post-pone death; to fail to do these things would be inhuman. In Western society, we turn above all to the medical profession for help, and the doctors who treat us belong to a profession that dates back to Hippocrates, the ancient Greek who, some 2,500 years ago, founded a tradition of medical education that continues uninterrupted to the present day. Yet the striking thing about the Hippocratic tradition of medicine is that, for all but the last hundred years, the therapies it relied on must have done (in so far as they acted on the body, not the mind) more harm than good. For some two thousand years, from the first century BC until the mid-nineteenth century, the main therapy used by doctors was bloodletting (usually opening a vein in the arm with a special knife called a lancet, a process called phlebotomy or venesection; but also sometimes cupping and leeching), which weakened and even killed patients.

Moreover medicine became more not less dangerous over time: nineteenth-century hospitals killed mothers in childbirth because doctors (trained to consider themselves scientists) unwittingly spread infections from mother to mother on their hands. Mothers and infants had been much safer in previous centuries when their care had been entrusted to informally trained midwives. For 2,400 years patients have believed that doctors were doing them good; for 2,300 years they were wrong.

I think it is fair to say that historians of medicine have had difficulty facing up to this fact. Historians of medicine are a diverse group, with widely differing views, but in general they no longer write about progress, and so they no longer seek to distinguish good medicine from bad. Indeed they try to avoid what they think of as anachronistic evaluations: 'only the most dyed-in-the-wool Whig history still polarizes the past in terms of confrontations between saints and sinners, heroes and villains', wrote Roy Porter (1946–2002, the greatest medical historian of his generation) in 1989. This book, on the other hand, is directly concerned with progress in medicine: what made it possible, and why it was so long postponed. To talk about progress is to talk about discoveries and innovation, and about obstacles and resistance: it is inevitably to talk about heroes and villains, if not about saints and sinners. This book, therefore, is written against the grain of contemporary historical writing.

There is a particular reason for writing about progress in medicine now. In recent years the medical profession has discovered what it calls 'evidence-based medicine'—that is, medicine that can be shown to work. This is the first history of medicine properly to acknowledge that most medicine, even into the present day, has not been evidence-based, and indeed that it did not work. If the story I tell in this book is very often one of failure not success that is because we have begun to redefine success, which means we are now in a position to rethink the history of medicine.

Recognizing how late and limited medical progress has been makes the progress that has taken place even more remarkable. So this book is also about the process whereby we have at long last learnt to preserve life and health. Here I have tried to concentrate on the big picture: the first successful operation on appendicitis took place, as best we can tell, in 1737; in Britain the first successful caesarean section, in which both mother and baby survived, had been performed by the end of the eighteenth century; but until 1865, when Joseph Lister, working in a Glasgow hospital, first demonstrated the principles of antiseptic surgery on a young boy with a compound fracture of the tibia, such operations were bound to be almost always fatal. With Lister there begins a new era in medicine, made possible by the triumph of germ theory, and the third part of this book examines the incredible revolution in medicine that began in 1865.

When I use phrases like 'until 1865' or 'a new era' I am using a sort of shorthand. There was considerable resistance to Lister's innovations, and they were slow to win acceptance. Despite the fact that antiseptic surgery helped consolidate a germ theory of disease, it was to be thirty years before a cure was found for any major infectious disease. The new era is separated from the old by a lengthy period of transition, from antiseptic surgery to penicillin, from 1865 to 1941, not by a single event, Lister's first antiseptic operation.

Moreover Lister's innovations made possible new types of bad medicine. For the first time it was possible to operate on the abdomen, and some surgeons proceeded to happily chop out bits and pieces (an appendix here, a colon there) not because they were infected, but because they might one day become infected—the historian Ann Dally has called this 'fantasy surgery'. These operations never became the norm, but tonsillectomies did, and we now know they did more harm than good. Worse still, the decision as to whose tonsils should be removed was not remotely rational. Of 1,000 11-year-old children in New York in 1934, 61 per cent had had tonsillectomies.

> The remaining 39 percent were subjected to examination by a group of physicians, who selected 45 percent of these for tonsillectomy and rejected the rest. The rejected children were re-examined by another group of physicians, who recommended tonsillectomy for 46 per cent of those remaining after the first examination. When the rejected children were examined a third time, a similar percentage was selected for tonsillectomy so that after three examinations only sixty-five children remained who had not been recommended for tonsillectomy. These subjects were not further examined because the supply of examining physicians ran out.

Clearly the decision as to who should have a tonsillectomy was entirely arbitrary. This was bad medicine alive and well in the 1930s.

I do not want to suggest that everything changed in 1865. But 1865 marks the moment when real progress first began in medical therapy, and, however imperfectly and haltingly, progress has continued since then. 1865 marks a turning point, not a transformation; by 1950 medicine had acquired a genuine capacity to extend life. This claim, that modern medicine works, is not I think really contentious. It once would have been. Between 1976, when Ivan Illich published *Limits to Medicine* and Thomas McKeown published *The Modern Rise of Population,* and 1995, when J. P. Bunker published an essay entitled

'Medicine Matters After All', there was a serious body of intellectual opinion which held that medicine had made no real difference to life expectancy, that the achievements of modern medicine were just as illusory as the achievements of ancient medicine. Now the balance of the argument has shifted: it is easy to exaggerate the extent to which medicine matters, but it would be strange to claim that it achieves nothing of any significance, and 1865 usefully marks the moment at which doctors began to be able to save lives.

Lister became a qualified doctor in 1854; the moment of his entry into the profession was marked, we may imagine, by his taking the Hippocratic Oath. The oath was written by Hippocrates when, in c.425 BC, he began to provide a medical education to people who were not members of his immediate family. Or at least this is what we are told by Galen, a Greek doctor who practised in Rome six hundred years later, and whose writings were, for 1,400 years, regarded, in both Islamic and Christian countries, as the ultimate authorities on all medical questions. A few years ago I watched with pride as my daughter took the Hippocratic Oath in Glasgow. There is something dizzying about the idea of a ritual that has survived for 2,500 years, while paganism has given way to monotheism, the mathematics of Pythagoras to the mathematics of Einstein, the technology of Archimedes to that of Werner von Braun, the Greek city state to the modern nation state.

The true story of the Hippocratic Oath is a bit more complicated. It almost certainly was written by Hippocrates. Scribonius Largus (c. AD 1–50) describes the oath being administered in his day; we have an Egyptian papyrus copy from c. AD 275. This evidence is so fragmentary that it suggests that the oath was not routinely employed in the education of doctors in the classical world, and it was certainly not regularly administered in the Middle Ages. We first find it being administered in a medical school in Wittenberg in Germany in 1508, and it first becomes part of a graduation ceremony in Montpellier in France in 1804. During the nineteenth century some European and American medical schools administered the oath, but many did not: I don't know if Lister took the oath or not. As late as 1928 only 19 per cent of American medical schools administered the oath; and it is only after the Second World War that the oath (in its various modernized forms) began to be administered almost universally. Nevertheless the oath effectively symbolizes the unbroken intellectual tradition descending from Hippocrates into the nineteenth century and, thanks to the conservatism of the medical profession, beyond. Even where continuity is an illusion (as it is in the case of the oath), not a reality, doctors have wanted to foster a sense of continuity. Or at least they have until very recently: the new move to problem-based learning, where medical students no longer attend lectures, means that in the future medical knowledge will cease to be presented as a body of information which has accumulated over time. Soon medical graduates will be taking the Hippocratic Oath without knowing who Hippocrates was.

In ancient Greece and Rome, throughout the world of Islam from the ninth century until the twentieth century (there were still 'Ionian' doctors practising ancient Greek medicine in Iraq in the 1970s, and I imagine there are still some today), in Western Europe from 1100 until the mid-nineteenth century, to be a doctor was not just to take one's place in a tradition descending from Hippocrates, it was to employ the therapies recommended by Hippocrates (although later generations were to place much more emphasis on bloodletting than Hippocrates himself had done). The standard editions of Hippocrates and Galen date to the moment when that tradition was coming to an end: 1839–61 in the case of Hippocrates, with an important English translation, 1849; 1821–33 in the case of Galen, with an important French translation, 1854–6. In the 1850s, when Lister went to university, Hippocrates and Galen were still part of every doctor's education.

1861, when the standard edition of Hippocrates was completed, is, as we shall see, an important date, the date of Pasteur's first major publication in germ theory and so (at least according to conventional accounts) the key moment in the founding of modern medicine. In 1846 the American J. R. Coxe could write of Hippocrates and Galen: 'the names of both these great men are familiar to our ears, as though they were the daily companions of our medical researches'. That daily companionship was to come to an end within a few years, but it had been so long-enduring, so constant, so intimate that nobody foresaw its end, and nobody celebrated its death. Hippocratic medicine had no funeral, no memorial, no obituary. Instead there was an almost wilful determination to pretend that modern medicine was a natural development from Hippocratic medicine, that Hippocrates could still be the doctor's daily companion.

At least until the 1860s there was a continuous tradition of Hippocratic medicine, and for century after century patients turned to their doctors to be cured. For two and a quarter millennia doctors insisted that medicine was a science that saved lives. But there were critics from the very beginning. An ancient work called *The Science of Medicine*, which dates to *c*.375 BC, is the first defence of Hippocratic medicine against its critics. The philosopher Heraclitus, for example, said that doctors tormented the sick, and were just as bad as the diseases they claimed to cure. It was Heraclitus, not the author of *The Science of Medicine*, who had the better argument, for Hippocratic medicine was incapable of fulfilling its promises. This should be obvious, but modern commentators are unable to admit this simple fact. They persist in treating *The Science of Medicine* as if it were a defence of science against quackery and superstition, rather than what in reality it is, a defence of quackery against justified scepticism. They seem to feel that the reputation of modern medicine is somehow at stake in this defence of ancient medicine, and that our idea of science is somehow the same as that of the ancient Greeks.

It is worth stressing that Hippocratic doctors were familiar with what we might think of as genuinely scientific and technological ways of thinking. A number of texts survive which the ancients attributed to Hippocrates; many were certainly written not by him but by his pupils, but amongst those with the best claim to have been written by Hippocrates himself is a work called *Fractures*, evidently written for the education of doctors in the fifth century BC. Its author explains how to make metal rods with which to force displaced broken bones back into place.

> One should use these, while extension is going on, to make leverage . . .
> just as if one would lever up violently a stone or log. This is a great help, if

the irons are suitable and the leverage used properly; for of all the apparatus contrived by men these three are the most powerful in action—
the wheel and axle, the lever and the wedge. Without some one, indeed,
or all of these, men accomplish no work requiring great force. This
lever method, then, is not to be despised, for the bones will be reduced
thus or not at all. If, perchance, the upper bone over-riding the other
affords no suitable hold for the lever, but being pointed, slips past, one
should cut a notch in the bone to form a secure lodgment for the lever.

This was a perfectly effective technology, well-grounded in theory;
but Hippocratic doctors persisted in defending bloodletting and
cauterization as if they were just as reliable as the application of a lever
to a stone or a log.

I have deliberately introduced the term 'technology' because I
want to stress that medicine, at least since Hippocrates, has always
been a technology, a set of techniques used to act on the material
world, in this case the physical condition of the patient's body. With
technologies it is perfectly legitimate, and not at all anachronistic, to
talk about progress. Thus a steam engine is a technology for turning
heat into propulsion. Progress in the design of steam engines means
either that greater propulsive force is obtained, or the same force is
obtained more efficiently. The definition of progress is internal to the
technology itself. In the case of medicine, progress means that pain is
alleviated, periods of sickness are shortened, and/or death is postponed. Hippocrates would have recognized this to be progress, so
would Lister, so would Richard Doll, the man who discovered that
smoking causes lung cancer. To ask if there is progress in medicine is
not to ask an illegitimate question, as it might be, for example, to ask if
there is progress in philosophy or poetry.

Hippocrates thought that he could alleviate pain, shorten sickness,
and postpone death. We now know that (in so far as his techniques
acted on the body not the mind) he was wrong. Studies in the nineteenth century, when Hippocratic therapies were finally coming
under attack, showed that when the standard Hippocratic therapies
were employed against broncho-pulmonary infections, mortality
was increased by about two-thirds. Hippocratic medicine was bad
medicine in that it killed when it claimed to cure.

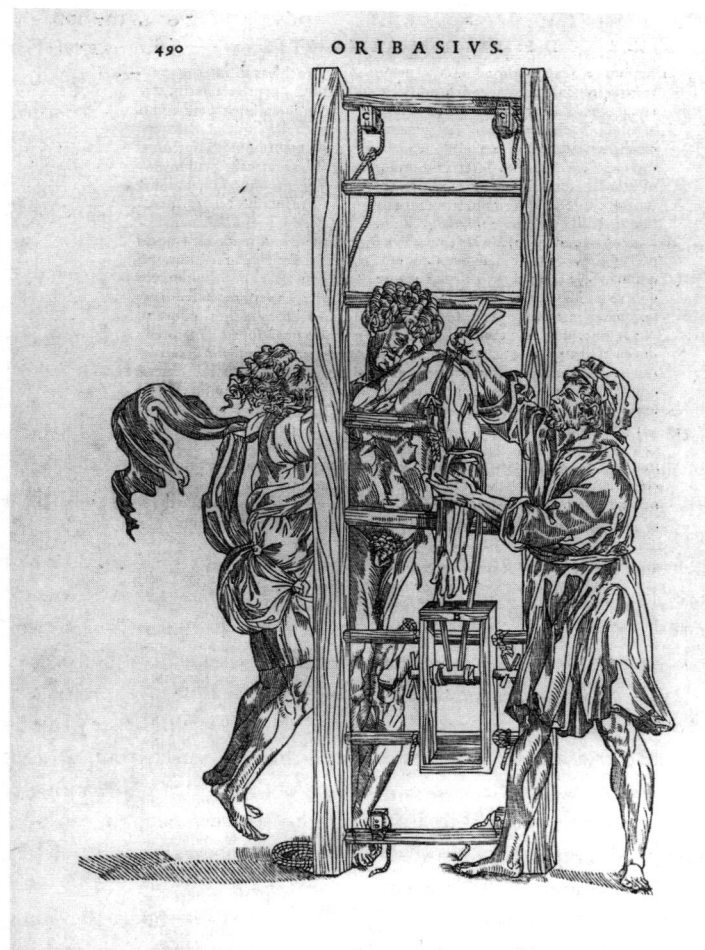

2. This woodcut, reproduced from Guido Guidi, *Opera Varia* (Lyons, 1599), first appears in 1544. It accompanies a text by the fourth-century Byzantine medical writer Oribasius. Hippocrates' *Fractures* is included in the same volume.

Of course Hippocrates did not know this, and he had no idea corresponding to our concept of an infectious disease. For Hippocrates no two illnesses were exactly alike; because illness was a disorder of a particular body each person's illnesses were to some degree idiosyncratic. Before you can start measuring the success of a therapy you need to start lumping particular occurrences of illness together. There are various ways in which you can come to do this. One is by recognizing that illnesses can be spread from one person to another—that the illness I have today is the very same one that you had yesterday. Most of the first claims that the effectiveness of therapies could be measured were directed at curing contagious diseases, and depended on the prior development of a concept of contagion.

But there are other ways of getting to the same result. Thomas Sydenham (1624–89), an English doctor and friend of John Locke, thought that Hippocrates had had a vital insight when he had seen that at certain times of year, in certain places, lots of people got very similar diseases. Sydenham did not believe in contagion, but he did believe that one could produce what he called 'an accurate history of diseases'. For too long people had thought of disease as 'but a confused and disordered effort of Nature, thrown down from her proper state, and defending herself in vain', but diseases had their own patterns and their own orderliness. Sydenham, like theorists of contagion, had come to think of diseases as if they fell into certain distinct species, just as (to use his comparison) plants did. Later generations of English doctors revered him as 'the English Hippocrates' because he had refounded medicine as a study, not of patients and their disorders, but of diseases and their regularities.

From this point it becomes easy, in principle, to compare therapies, and decide if one is better than another at alleviating pain, shortening illness, and postponing death—Sydenham claimed to have brought about a great improvement in the treatment of smallpox (even though he did not recognize it as a contagious disease). Other doctors had bled smallpox victims, covered them with hot blankets, and given them warming drinks, despite the fact that they were suffering from a fever. Sydenham thought this could lead to boiling of the blood, brain-fever, and death. He cooled his patients, gave them cool liquids, and, naturally, bled them, though only moderately. His patients were certainly more comfortable, and may well have got better faster. For other conditions, however, his therapies were entirely orthodox. He believed, for example in treating a cough, of whatever sort (he was well aware there were different sorts of cough), with bleeding and (often repeated) purges (laxatives to induce diarrhoea).

In Sydenham's day, people were beginning the first systematic study of life expectancies, based on the London 'bills of mortality', which recorded the cause of death for everyone who died in London. As we shall see, the new intellectual tools were being assembled which would eventually make it possible to evaluate therapies and measure progress in medicine. The more this was done, the more it became apparent that traditional remedies were defective. Foucault gives the example of an early nineteenth-century doctor who abandoned all the traditional therapies. He was aware of 2,000 species of disease, and treated each and every one of them with quinine. Now quinine, a drug that was new in the seventeenth century, really does work against malaria. Its great advantage in use against the other 1,999 conditions is that (unlike traditional Hippocratic remedies) it does little harm.

Although Hippocrates had no way of knowing it, his technology was defective. Hippocratic medicine was not a science, but a fantasy of science; and in this it is much more like astrology than it is like Ptolemaic astronomy (the classical account which placed the earth at the centre of the cosmos, with the sun and planets rotating around it), for classical astronomy worked rather well as a method of predicting the movements of bodies in the heavens. But where modern astronomy founded itself in the rejection of astrology, where the astrologers were thrown out of the universities by the astronomers, modern medicine incorporated the Hippocratic tradition and the Hippocratic profession. Where the history of astronomy was long written as if it had nothing to do with astrology, so that modern historians have had to rediscover the fact that astronomy and astrology were once one and the same thing, history of medicine has been written as if it has everything to do with Hippocrates, so that the historian now has to discover the fact that Hippocratic medicine was not itself a science, but a fantasy of science. The whole of medicine before 1865 was caught up in a fantasy world.

One reason for this appearance of continuity, this peculiar insistence that the history of medicine begins with Hippocrates, not with Pasteur or with Lister, is that in medicine the astrologers turned into astronomers, the Hippocratic doctors turned into scientific doctors. But there is another reason, and that is that the new doctors kept on doing the equivalent of casting horoscopes. Until the invention of penicillin in 1941 there was very little doctors could do about most infections; even the new science left them virtually powerless in the face of disease. They had no alternative but to keep up the age-old pretence that medicine had something useful to offer, when for the most part what it offered was a ritual, a rite, a performance, a show. Doctors did not cure patients; rather they helped them contain their anxieties, which is an important undertaking in itself. But the age-old pretence that they could do more than this still affects the way in which we write about the history of medicine, and prevents us from thinking straight about progress in medicine.

The medical revolution of the second half of the nineteenth century meant that soon textbooks were no longer restatements of the teachings of Hippocrates and Galen; but the notion that medicine was a long-standing profession, that it had an ancient tradition, was preserved in the face of change. Just as the medical profession survived surprisingly unchanged, so too our language continues to reflect the beliefs and practices of an earlier age. When I say my blood boils; when I admit I'm hysterical; when I assume that red-headed people are hot-blooded or complain that someone is cold-blooded or ill-humoured; when I say someone is phlegmatic; when I listen to the song 'My Melancholy Baby', I'm thinking in terms which once made sense as part of a coherent and subtle system of belief. Our language is littered with the flotsam and jetsam of a vast historical catastrophe, the collapse of ancient medicine, which has left us with half-understood turns of phrase that we continue to use because metaphorical habits have an extraordinary capacity for endurance. It has also left us with a vocabulary which seems so completely modern that we scarcely even realize that we have inherited it from the ancient Greeks: apoplexy, arthritis, asthma, cancer, coma, cholera, emphysema, haemorrhoid, hepatitis, herpes, jaundice, leprosy, nephritis, ophthalmia, paraplegia, pleurisy, pneumonia, spasm, tetanus, typhus amongst the diseases; artery, muscle, nerve and vein amongst the parts of the body. The history of ancient medicine is still, though only just, a part of our own history.

The whole enterprise of the history of medicine has been vitiated by its inability to take seriously the extent to which medicine was, until 1865, an impossible, a misconceived project. Before contemporary history of medicine (roughly speaking, history of medicine since 1973), medical history was presented as a grand narrative of progress, and indeed there is some logic to such a narrative as long as one thinks of medicine as a body of knowledge or a science, not as a technology for treating illness. The first historian (he resisted even the word 'historian', preferring at one point 'archaeologist', at another 'genealogist') to break with the grand narrative of progress was Michel Foucault, whose *The Birth of the Clinic: An Archaeology of Medical Perception* appeared in 1963 in French and 1973 in English. But Foucault thought that modern medicine began in 1816, with the pathological anatomy of François Broussais, that modern medicine could be identified with a particular way of looking at patients' bodies, not, as I will argue, with the germ theory of disease. So his book was not about progress in medicine at all, at least not in the sense of medicine understood as a technology. Broussais was no better at curing diseases than Hippocrates had been, even if he preferred letting blood by applying leeches to the body (often to the anus) rather than by using a lancet to slice into a vein, as Galen would have done. Actually, as we shall see, the story Foucault tells in *The Birth of the Clinic* is best understood, not as the story of the birth of modern medicine, but as the story of the final crisis of ancient medicine.

A central claim of this book is that one of the most interesting things about medicine is that it works, and that we therefore need to study progress in medicine. We can only think about medical progress if we start with the long tradition of medical failure. We need to begin with bad medicine if we are to understand better medicine. We need, quite consciously and deliberately, to engage in what Porter called a polarization of the past. We need to think about the obstacles to progress, about the villains as well as the heroes.

When my daughter was 8, some twenty years ago, I bought her a large pop-up book called *The Body*. It contained illustrations of bones, muscles, and nerves, and of organs such as the heart and the uterus. Back then, before computer simulation, there was something mesmerizing about the crude three-dimensionality of folded paper. We both found it fascinating. Thinking I was being a good parent, I took the opportunity the various images of sexual organs presented of explaining, in the simplest terms, sexual reproduction. My daughter was puzzled. The next day she came back from school and said she had discussed the matter with her friends. My theories were quite mistaken. No physical contact between the mummy and the daddy was needed to make a baby. She had consulted the ultimate authority, her peer group, and that was the end of the matter.

At the time I thought my attempt to teach my daughter elementary biology had been a hopeless failure, but since she has now grown up to be a doctor, perhaps I achieved more than I realized. At any rate, I learnt a great deal from that experience, and this book has its origin in that conversation. For I had been educated on John Locke and John Stuart Mill. I took it for granted that in an open argument good ideas would always defeat bad ideas; this was what made progress possible. I assumed that I only had to explain modern science to her in order for her to believe in it. I had no understanding of why someone might reject an unfamiliar and unwelcome idea.

However, the real world is not the world of Locke and Mill. There was something fundamentally wrong with my idea of how knowledge is transmitted from one person to another. Bad ideas often triumph over good: we will see a striking example of this when we look at the history of scurvy. Peer-group pressure often halts progress in its tracks. Despite the brilliant work of philosophers and historians of science (including historians of medicine), no one has really worked out how to write a history that takes account of this. We know how to write histories of discovery and progress, but not how to write histories of stasis, of delay, of digression. We know how to write about the delight of discovery, but not about attachment to the old and resistance to the new. We know how to write about drug patents and about the growth of new industries, but not about the ways in which economic interests can obstruct change. We know how to write about successful treatments and lives saved, but not about worthless therapies and lives lost. We know how to write old-fashioned histories of progress, although for the most part we choose not to do so. Because we only know how to tell one half of the story, the story we could tell is so obviously unsatisfactory that (if we are professional historians) we usually choose not to tell it.

Many years ago, in 1932, a famous historian, Herbert Butterfield, wrote an attack on narratives of progress called *The Whig Interpretation of History*. Butterfield's immediate target was a view of English history that saw it as being about the progress of liberty—a view invented by the Whig party in the eighteenth century. As a result 'Whig history' has become the label for any anachronistic history of progress, and the self-confessed 'dyed-in-the-wool Whig historian' (to quote once again Roy Porter in one of the epigraphs to this book) has become an extinct species. Butterfield seems to have recognized that historians were bound to slip into such narratives, and happily slipped into them himself in many of his short books on big subjects, such as his book entitled *The Origins of Modern Science*. The alternative, he thought, was a sort of technical history that presented events as being the result of enormously complex processes, and described outcomes as being uncertain and unpredictable. Butterfield thought there were in effect two types of history: a bird's eye view, which surveyed the past from the point of view of the present, and was necessarily biased and ana-chronistic; and a worm's eye view, in which small things loomed large, and it was impossible to get one's bearings. Since Butterfield there has been a general agreement amongst historians that the best history is written from a worm's eye view—despite the fact that some problems only come into focus if one stands back and looks at the big picture.

Go into any good bookshop and you will discover that there is more than one type of medical history. Much history of medicine is written by doctors for doctors. It deals with the past from a doctor's point of view, not from a historian's. There are many books that survey the key discoveries in medical history. Several of these books contain a chapter on the invention of the stethoscope by René Laennec in 1816. Doctors still use stethoscopes, indeed one of the first things a medical student does is buy a stethoscope, and so the invention of the first stethoscope looks like an important step towards modern medicine. One of the first uses of the stethoscope was to improve the diagnosis of women suffering from phthisis. Where a doctor could not put his ear to a woman's chest as he could to a man's, he could put his stethoscope there and hear the characteristic sounds associated with phthisis. Phthisis no longer exists as a disease: we now call it tuberculosis because we think of it as an infectious disease caused by a specific micro-organism. The same sounds in a stethoscope that would once have led to a diagnosis of phthisis now leads to tests to confirm tuberculosis. But there is an important difference between our diagnosis of tuberculosis and Laennec's diagnosis of phthisis: we can cure tuberculosis (most of the time), while his patients died of phthisis—he died of it himself. Until 1865 (when Lister introduced antiseptic surgery) virtually all medical progress was of this sort. It enabled doctors to get better and better at prognosis, at predicting who would die, but it made no difference at all to therapeutics. It was a progress in science but not in technology.

We tend to assume that where there is progress in knowledge there is progress in therapy: for over the last hundred years the two have gone hand in hand. But before 1865 progress in knowledge rarely led to improvements in therapy. So we need a history of medicine that recognizes that progress can long be irrelevant (as in the case of the stethoscope). Nineteenth-century doctors could hear chest wheezes and heart murmurs through their stethoscopes; but there was no treatment for tuberculosis before 1942, and no effective heart surgery before 1948. Diagnosis was pointless without an effective therapy. Only once there was a treatment for tuberculosis did the stethoscope become a powerful tool. And this is one example of a much wider pattern. Much knowledge that was effectively useless at first became useful once new therapies began to be devised. The knowledge about human physiology and the diagnostic techniques that had been accumulated by doctors over time took on a new significance once they could be used to enable effective therapies; in that sense modern doctors have been able to draw on reserves of knowledge accumulated over centuries, just as modern astronomers could draw on the knowledge accumulated by astrologers.

The idea that progress in knowledge and progress in therapy are quite distinct may seem an obvious point, but it took me a long while to grasp it. When I started working on this book, my intention was to write a history of different ways of conceiving of the human body—in terms of the four humours (ancient and medieval medicine); as a mechanical system in which the heart functions as a bellows (the medicine of the scientific revolution); as a system of chemical interactions (nineteenth-century medicine); as a system for the replication of genes (twentieth-century medicine), and so forth. Each represented itself as an advance on its predecessors.

But then I recognized that there was a fundamental difference between ideas about the body and medical therapies. Between the sixteenth and the nineteenth centuries, ideas about the body changed fundamentally, but therapies changed very little. Bloodletting was the main medical therapy in 1500, 1800, and 1850. The discovery of the circulation of the blood (1628), of oxygen (1775), of the role of haemoglobin (1862) made no difference; the discoveries were adapted to the therapy rather than vice versa. Textbook histories of medicine make it hard to understand this because they emphasize change not continuity. And they just assume or assert that bloodletting was phased out early in the nineteenth century when in fact it continued long afterwards. Thus they try to elide a basic fact: if you look at therapy, not theory, then ancient medicine survived more or less intact into the middle of the nineteenth century and beyond.

Strangely, traditional medical practices—bloodletting, purging, inducing vomiting—had continued even while people's understanding of how the body worked underwent radical alteration. The new theories were set to work to justify the old practices. Venous and arterial blood, for example, were still thought about as if they were fundamentally different even after Harvey had shown that the one changed constantly into the other, and even after it became clear that the difference between them was that one contained oxygen and the

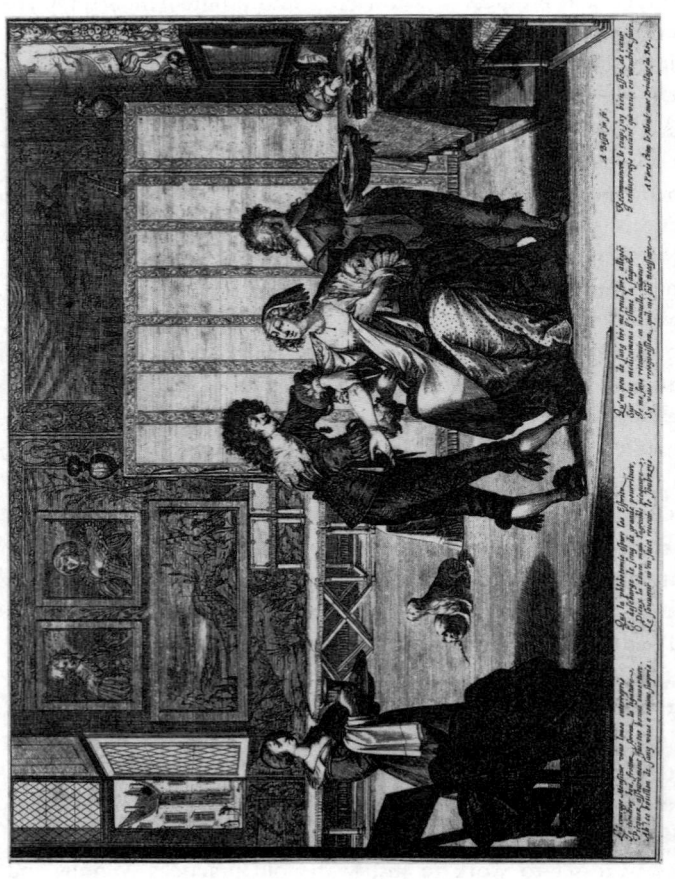

3. Abraham Bosse, *Bloodletting*, *c*.1635. This etching shows a doctor in seventeenth-century France tying the ligature around an aristocratic patient's arm before letting blood.

other did not. And this imaginary difference had to be preserved in order to justify the claim that letting venous blood could cure disease, while the letting of arterial blood was always to be avoided. It is because of this fundamental continuity in therapies and in theories of disease (bad air was thought to be the cause of epidemic disease in the mid-nineteenth century just as in the days of Hippocrates), even though theories of the body had undergone radical change, that I use the terms 'Hippocratic medicine' and 'traditional medicine' to cover not just the period when humoral theory was in the ascendant, but the whole period through to the rise of the germ theory of disease.

Having recognized that therapies stood still even while knowledge advanced, I had to face a deeply disturbing fact. Much of the new knowledge was founded on vivisection. This did not greatly worry me, I have to confess, for as long as I thought that all medical knowledge was useful knowledge. But how could you justify the suffering of Harvey's experimental animals when you realized that Harvey was no better at treating the sick than any other seventeenth-century doctor? As I worked on this book, I became more and more puzzled at the way in which standard medical histories ignored vivisection, which turned out to be absolutely central to the history of medicine. Vivisection, and even dissection, I realized were difficult and emotionally disturbing subjects, and one needed to face the fact that modern medicine had been born out of a series of activities that were both shocking and distressing. As long as I thought of medical history in terms of a continuing progress in knowledge, I could assume that dissection and vivisection were worth it; but once I realized that there was virtually no progress in therapy before 1865, I was bound to ask myself how one could justify mangling the dead and torturing the living.

And then I slowly became aware of a third problem. Histories of progress are written on the assumption that there is a logic of discovery. Once you discover α (say, germs), it is easy to discover β (say, antibiotics); without a theory of germs you will never discover antibiotics. A good example is Newton's theory of gravity. As long as the sun, the moon, the planets, and the stars were believed to circle around the earth it seemed obvious that there were different laws of movement on earth and in the heavens—here, natural movement was in a straight line, there it was in a circle; when, with the Copernican theory, the earth became a planet moving through the heavens, it became possible to ask if the same laws governed movement on earth and in the heavens. Copernicus is thus a precondition for Newton, and the discovery of gravity requires that one first surmount a number of major epistemological barriers, beginning with rejecting the evidence of one's own senses, which tell one that the earth stands still.

Once the epistemological barriers to a discovery have been overcome, the discovery itself ought to follow rapidly and fairly easily. The classic stories of discovery thus include priority disputes, such as whether Servetus discovered the circulation of the blood before Harvey. Or they include independent but almost simultaneous discoveries: Priestley and Scheele, for example, both discovered oxygen; Newton and Leibniz both discovered calculus; Cagniard-Latour and Schwann both discovered that yeast is animate. The logic of scientific discovery seems so strong that it either bears individuals along, or it makes individuals irrelevant. Pasteur said that his work was shaped by an inflexible logic, and one might assume that the same logic also shaped the work of his contemporaries. Pasteur published on putrefaction in 1863; Lister developed antiseptic surgery two years later, and stressed how closely his own discovery followed on Pasteur's work. Once Pasteur had discovered a vaccine for anthrax in 1881, the hunt for other vaccines was on. Once penicillin had been discovered in 1941, the hunt for other antibiotics was on.

But the more I looked for the logic of discovery, the more often it seemed to slip through my fingers. Harvey announced that the heart pumped blood through the arteries in 1628; yet the use of the tourniquet in amputations, which one would have thought was an absolutely elementary application of Harvey's theory, was first pioneered by Jean Louis Petit (1674–1750), roughly a century later. Leeuwenhoek saw what we would now loosely call germs, or more accurately bacteria, through his microscope in 1677; yet in 1820 microscopes had no place in medical research, and in 1881 the conflict between germ theorists and their opponents was only just entering its final phase. Penicillin was first discovered not in 1941 but in 1872. And so on.

What we need in cases such as these is a history, not of progress, but of delay; not of events, but of non-events; not of an inflexible logic but of a sloppy logic, not of overdetermination, but of underdetermination. And these cases, it turns out, are in medicine (at least until very recently) the norm, not the exceptions. To give a recent example, the discovery that bacteria (and not stress) cause stomach ulcers met with considerable resistance and was only generally accepted—and rewarded with the 2005 Nobel prize for medicine—after a prolonged delay: it is too soon to say whether this is now an exceptional case or not. Delay may have been, may still be, normal, but the reasons for it vary greatly.

Let me briefly take one example. Whenever our bodies are involved, our feelings and emotions, our hopes and fears, our delights and disgusts, are engaged. Medicine has often involved doing things to other people that you normally should not do—touching them, hurting them, cutting them open. Think for a moment what surgery was like before the invention of anaesthesia in 1842. Imagine amputating the limb of a patient who is screaming and struggling. Imagine training yourself to be indifferent to the patient's suffering, to be deaf to their screams. Imagine developing the strength to pin down the patient's thrashing body. Imagine learning how to be, as Ambroise Paré, the great sixteenth-century surgeon who pioneered the tying off of blood vessels when performing amputations, put it, 'resolute and merciless'. Imagine taking pride, above all, in the speed with which you wield the knife, in never having to pause for thought or breath: speed was essential, for the shock of an operation could itself be a major factor in bringing about the patient's death.

Now think about this: in 1795 a doctor discovered that inhaling nitrous oxide killed pain, and the fact was published and discussed. Nitrous oxide was used as a fairground amusement; there was no mystery about its properties. Yet no surgeon experimented with this, the first anaesthetic, nor with carbon dioxide, which Henry Hill Hickman was using as a general anaesthetic on animals from 1824. The use of anaesthetics was pioneered not by surgeons but by humble dentists, not in London, or Paris, or Berlin, the centres of medical research, but first in Rochester, NY, and then in Boston. One of the first practitioners of painless dentistry, Horace Wells, was driven to suicide by the hostility of the medical profession. When anaesthesia was first employed in Europe, in London in 1846, it was called a 'Yankee dodge'. In other words, practising anaesthesia felt like cheating. Most of the characteristics the surgeon had developed—the indifference, the strength, the pride, the sheer speed—were suddenly irrelevant.

Why did it take fifty years to invent anaesthesia? Any answer has to recognize the emotional investment surgeons had made in becoming a certain sort of person with a certain set of skills and the difficulty of abandoning that self-image. Interestingly, the first European to adopt the Yankee dodge was the surgeon who had least to fear from the accusation of cheating: Robert Liston, the man who best embodied the traditional skills of the surgeon, the man who worked faster than anyone else.

The history of medicine has to be something more than just a history of knowledge; it also has to be a history of emotion. And this is difficult because our own emotions are involved. The truth is that historians do not like thinking about what surgery was like before anaesthesia. They too deafen themselves to the patients' cries. The result is that we never actually hear what we need to hear: because we have not listened out for the screams, we never hear the eerie silence that fell over operating tables in the 1850s.

If we turn to other discoveries we find that they too have the puzzling feature of unnecessary delay we have just seen in the case of anaesthesia. So if we do start looking at progress we find we actually need to tell a story of delay as well as a story of discovery, and in order to make sense of these delays we need to turn away from the inflexible logic of discovery and look at other factors: the role of the emotions, the limits of imagination, the conservatism of institutions, to name just three. If you want to think about what progress really means, then you need to imagine what it was like to have become so accustomed to the screams of patients that they seemed perfectly natural and normal; so accustomed to them that you could read with interest about nitrous oxide, could go to a fairground and try it out, and never even imagine that it might have a practical application. To think about progress, you must first understand what stands in the way of progress—in this case, the surgeon's pride in his work, his professional training, his expertise, his sense of who he is.

Anaesthetics made the work of surgery easier. They were no threat to surgeons' incomes. At first sight surgeons had everything to gain and nothing to lose from the discovery of pain relief. And indeed, from 1846, anaesthesia established itself with great speed. Yet it is clear from the inexplicable delay, from the extraordinary hostility expressed towards its inventors, from the use of the phrase 'Yankee dodge', that there was something at stake, some obstacle to be overcome. That obstacle was the surgeons' own image of themselves.

Since this book argues that real medicine begins with germ theory, at its heart there is a most puzzling historical non-event: the long delay that took place between the discovery of germs and the triumph of germ theory. It's fairly easy to find names for things that happen—the Scientific Revolution, the Great War. It's much harder to name a non-event, but non-events can be every bit as important as events. Historians regularly insist that to understand the past one must approach it as if one did not know what was going to happen next. But, despite this, they are very reluctant to take seriously the idea that things might have happened differently. The standard view is that when important things don't happen it is because they couldn't possibly have happened. Thus the great biologist François Jacob, in *The Logic of Living Things*, argues that eighteenth-century biologists could not solve the intellectual problems presented by sexual reproduction: which is why most of them accepted preformationism, the claim that every future human being was already present in Eve's ovaries.

But Jacob recognizes that another problem that exercised eighteenth-century scientists is rather different: most of them believed in the spontaneous generation of micro-organisms, but there was no logical reason for them to think that micro-organisms were different from organisms visible to the naked eye. The issues raised by spontaneous generation were nothing like as conceptually puzzling and problematic as those raised by sexual reproduction, and yet until they were resolved there could be no satisfactory germ theory of disease, and therefore no real progress in medicine.

Belief in spontaneous generation was not sustained by some insuperable intellectual obstacle. We must look elsewhere for an explanation of its endurance—to the technical problems associated with experiments to disprove spontaneous generation, certainly, but also to a profound reluctance to accept that what one could see through a microscope could have any relevance to our own lives. Sydenham, for example, who was as we have seen one of the first to have a modern concept of disease, acknowledged that the key processes that took place within the body must take place on a minute scale. You might think he would immediately have reached for a microscope in order to study them. But no. Writing in 1668, when the first living creature invisible to the naked eye had just been discovered, he dismissed the microscope as irrelevant. How could one hope to dissect such a minute creature and identify its internal organs? No microscope, he said, could possibly see anything so small. Consequently the microscope could not enable us to see any important process going on in our own bodies. The enquiry was abandoned as pointless before it was even begun. I do not think one can call this a rational response, so one has to assume Sydenham was in part unconscious of his own motives in rejecting the microscope.

As long as people assumed one could learn nothing of importance by looking through a microscope the debate over the spontaneous generation of micro-organisms was an intellectual backwater. The microscope became a recognized tool for research in 1830; by 1837 the key experiment disproving spontaneous generation had been performed. If Sydenham and people like him had been willing to reach for their microscopes, the issue could have been resolved at least a hundred years earlier.

In saying this I am passing judgement on Sydenham for failing to understand the potential of the microscope. This is inevitable because there is no such thing as an impartial account of the debate provoked by a scientific discovery. When Oliver Wendell Holmes, giving a farewell address to students and colleagues on his retirement from

Harvard University in 1882, referred to 'the dark ages of medicine' when bloodletting was the cure for every disease (the quotation is one of the epigraphs to this book), he had earned the right to use such strong language, because he was talking about the medicine in which he had been educated as a young man, and during his career he had fought a series of battles to bring light into darkness. But any historian of the transformation in medicine during Holmes's career also needs to decide whether they are for or against bloodletting. In the disputes in which Holmes had been involved the two sides had disagreed about what the relevant information was, and about how to interpret it: we have known to expect this since Thomas Kuhn's *Structure of Scientific Revolutions* (1962). Since their points of view are radically different, you have to choose between them. You have to take sides.

I first began to understand this when I read a wonderful book, from which I have taken another epigraph, John Tyndall's *Floating Matter in the Air* (1882). Tyndall was at the heart of the intellectual revolution associated with the triumph of germ theory. In 1875 he carried out a delicate series of experiments designed to prove the truth of germ theory and disprove the alternative, spontaneous generation. The experiments worked perfectly, and he published the results with pride. A year later he tried to repeat the experiments, and over and over again what he seemed to produce was evidence of spontaneous generation. He just could not get the results he had obtained only a year before. One might think that Tyndall should have changed his mind in the light of the new evidence. Instead he treated the new evidence as an obstacle to be overcome. He refused to give up, he refused to give in, he was determined not to be defeated. And this, every scientist would now say, was the right choice. There can be no impartial account of Tyndall's refusal to accept the result of his own experiments, of his stubborn persistence in face of the evidence: what one makes of it depends entirely on whether one is a proponent of germ theory or of spontaneous generation.

So don't be misled by the title of this book. This is neither an attack on the medical profession nor an indictment of modern medicine. When I was young, doctors twice saved my life: I have the scars to prove it. More recently, a plastic surgeon performed a wonderful operation on my right hand, on which I'd lost the use of two fingers. I'm all in favour of good medicine—but the subject of good medicine is inseparable from the subject of bad medicine. To think about one, you need to be able to think about the other, and of the two subjects, bad medicine is both the less explored and by far the larger. Before 1865 all medicine was bad medicine, that is to say, it did far more harm than good. But 1865 did not usher in a new era of good medicine. For the three paradoxes of progress—ineffectual progress, immoral progress, progress postponed—are still at work. They may not work quite as powerfully now as they did before 1865, but they work more powerfully than we are prepared to acknowledge. There has been progress; but not nearly as much as most of us believe.

In the final chapter of the book I will try to measure the extent of the progress that has taken place. I think most readers will be surprised to discover just how limited the achievements of modern medicine are. And, as we shall see, the paradoxes of progress do not cover the full range of problems we encounter in modern medicine. There is, for example, iatrogenesis, where medical intervention itself creates conditions that need to be treated, a particular case of doing harm when trying to do good. But other subjects, I want to stress now, lie outside the scope of this book, important though they are. This book is not concerned with plain malpractice. There have always been incompetent, careless, and even malevolent doctors, but what I am concerned with in this book is the medical profession at its best. My subject is the bad medicine that was honestly believed to be good medicine. Second, this book is concerned only with physical, not with mental disease: the story of bad psychiatry would require at least a volume to itself. Third, this book is concerned with medicine in Western Europe and America. There were rapid advances after 1865 in the understanding and treatment of tropical diseases, and a chapter on typhoid or malaria might not have been out of place. But I have chosen to concentrate on medicine in those countries which first benefited from a sustained increase in life expectancy, for they are the countries in which we may best assess the impact of medical progress. But first, I suggest, before we study progress, we must make an effort to understand failure.

I. THE HIPPOCRATIC TRADITION

1

HIPPOCRATES AND GALEN

As we have seen, medicine begins with Hippocrates. For more than two thousand years doctors have revered his memory, yet we know so little about him that some have dismissed him as a mythical figure. The truth is that we are not absolutely sure whether Hippocrates existed or whether later doctors invented him. Hippocrates of Cos (a tiny island in the Mediterranean) apparently lived from around 460 to around 375 BC. Later generations believed some sixty works by him survived, but modern scholars argue that these works were written over a period of two hundred years or so, and that it is quite possible that none of them are actually by Hippocrates. It is not difficult, however, to identify a number of respects in which the first Hippocratics represent an entirely new approach to medicine.

First, Hippocrates and his immediate followers insisted that disease always had a natural, rather than a supernatural origin. There was no point, then, in relying on religious ceremonies, prayers, or charms to cure disease. Instead the doctor had to identify the cause of the disease and work to counteract it. Their starting assumption was that everything had a natural cause. Second, the Hippocratic authors were committed to a programme of careful observation. One set of books, the *Epidemics*, is a series of case studies of individual patients and particular outbreaks of disease. Observation extended, for example, to a very careful study of the development of the chicken embryo in the egg, conducted by opening an egg each day for twenty days, for the light it might cast on the development of the human embryo. Hippocrates and his successors established a tradition of medical observation and education that descends unbroken to the present day.

For Hippocrates and his contemporaries there were two fundamental branches to medicine. First there was the type of medicine that involved hands-on manipulation of the body: lancing a boil, setting a bone, reducing a dislocation. They had considerable skills at dealing with injuries, which were common in warfare and gymnastics. When Pausanias visited Delphi in the second century BC he reported that 'Among the votive offerings to Apollo was a representation in bronze of a man's body in an advanced state of decay, with the flesh already fallen off and nothing left but the bones. The Delphians said that it was an offering of Hippocrates the physician.' Pausanius obviously had difficulty describing this strange sculpture, but it sounds very much like what we would call a skeleton (we will look at the history of the word later), a representation of the body ideal for teaching hands-on medicine.

Second, there was the type of medicine that was concerned with the inner workings of the body. The skeleton was envisaged as supporting a number of containers that were, at least in illness if not in health, full of fluid. In a work contemporary with Hippocrates we are told that:

> Every part of the body which is covered by flesh or muscle contains a cavity. Every separate organ, whether covered by skin or muscle, is hollow, and in health is filled with life-giving spirit; in sickness it is pervaded by unhealthy humours. The arms, for example, possess such a cavity, as do the thighs and legs. Even those parts which are relatively poorly covered with flesh contain such cavities. Thus the trunk is hollow and contains the liver, the skull contains the brain and the thorax the lungs. Thus the divisions of the body may be likened to a series of vessels, each containing within it various organs, some of which are harmful and some beneficial to their possessor.

These cavities were connected together in ways that now puzzle us. Thus the pupils of Hippocrates would let blood from the vein in the right elbow to relieve pain in the liver, and blood from the vein in the left elbow to relieve pain in the spleen because they believed these blood vessels were directly connected to these organs. At least this is how we would describe what they would do: they did not distinguish between veins and arteries, having a general term for blood vessels, and did not have a word for organs, using instead a word that means 'shapes'.

Hippocrates and his immediate successors shared two further assumptions. The first was that you should manage the conduct of daily life so that the right amount and type of food, drink, exercise, sleep and so forth encouraged health, and when disease set in you should try to counteract excess or deficiency—so they prescribed exercise for someone who rested too much, or dieting for someone who ate too much. This seems to be the original context in which the fundamental principle that opposites are cured by opposites—what the Middle Ages was to call the Law of Hippocrates—was first formulated.

Second, you could eliminate excess fluids from the body by inducing vomiting (using emetics), by inducing diarrhoea (using purgatives and enemas), or by letting blood. There were two classical methods of letting blood. The first was the cutting of a vein; the second was 'cupping' where the surface of the skin was scratched and a cup applied to it and a sucking force introduced, either by directly sucking air out of a hole in the base of the cup, or by first heating the cup and then letting it cool while attached to the body—this removed blood more slowly and cautiously than did venesection. Much later a third method was to be introduced: leeches were applied to suck blood from the body. The followers of Hippocrates also had an interest in cautery, the application of hot irons to parts of the body. These four forms of treatment (emetics, purgatives, bloodletting, and cautery) were to remain the fundamental therapies for almost two thousand years; three of the four were to remain the standard therapies for far longer than that. (Cautery was largely abandoned in the Renaissance, but Laennec, the inventor of the stethoscope, offered it to patients suffering from phthisis (tuberculosis), knowing that conventional remedies were ineffectual. He made 12 to 15 burns on the chest with an incandescent copper rod.) It seems likely that these procedures all predated Hippocrates: the Scythians practised cautery, and we have a Greek perfume bottle from c.475 BC which shows a doctor engaged in venesection, with a cupping bowl hanging on the wall behind him. What the Hippocratics provided was an account of why these therapies worked: it never occurred to them that they did not.

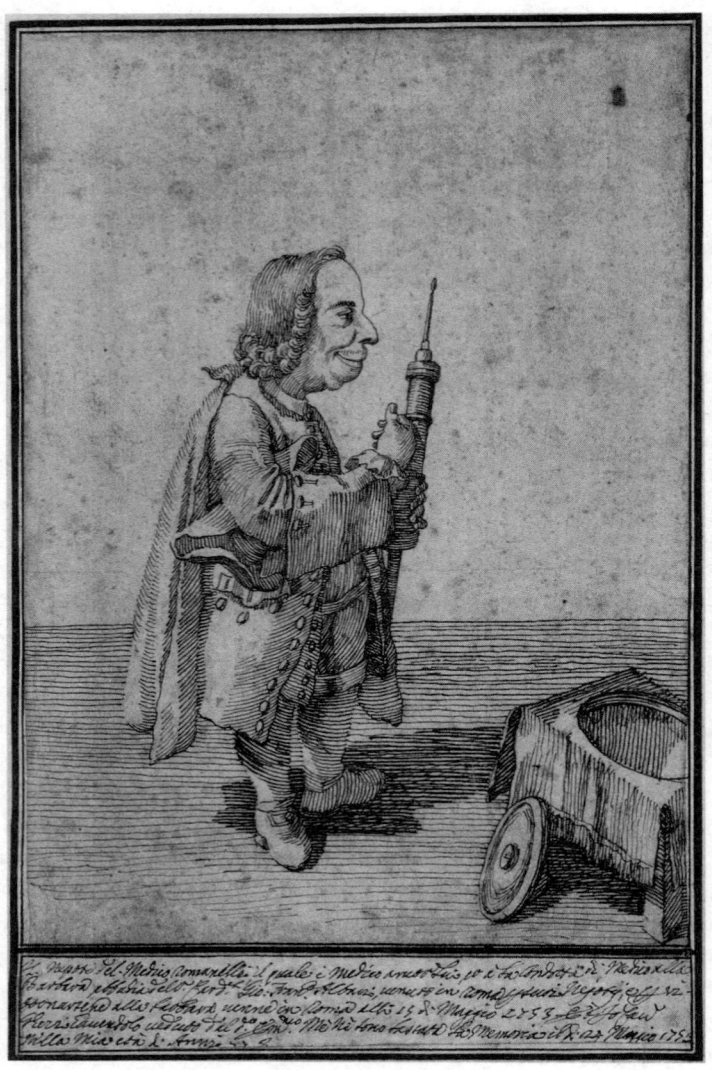

4. This eighteenth-century caricature, by Pier Leone Ghezzi, shows a Dr
Romanelli, who was employed by Cardinal Giovanni Francesco Albani.
He is holding an enema syringe.

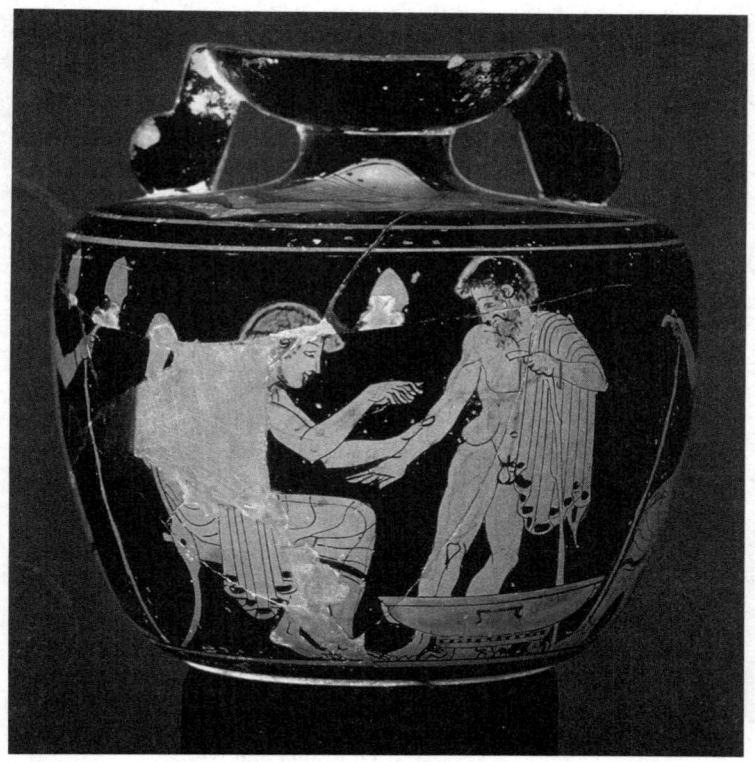

5. A Greek vase from c.475 BC showing a doctor's surgery.

All the Hippocratics shared a belief that the human body was an
integrated whole. In order to understand what was going on inside it
you had to study the fluids that came out of it (vomit, urine, blood,
phlegm, etc.), but it was assumed that a whole range of other indicators might serve as signs indicating internal processes. Here is a passage from a treatise called *Epidemics I* (c.410 BC) that is amongst those
preserved by later generations of doctors because they believed it to
be by Hippocrates himself. The author describes an outbreak of *causus*
(perhaps enteric fever) in the autumn. Those affected suffered from
fever, fits, insomnia, thirst, nausea, delirium, cold sweats, constipation,

and they passed urine 'which was black and fine'; death often occurred on the sixth day, or the eleventh, or the twentieth.

> The disease was very widespread. Of those who contracted it death was most common among youths, young men, men in the prime of life, those with smooth skins, those of a pallid complexion, those with straight hair, those with black hair, those with black eyes, those who had been given to violent and loose living, those with thin voices, those with rough voices, those with lisps and the choleric. Many women also succumbed to this malady.

Much of this seems irrelevant to us; and reading through this list it is hard for us to avoid the impression that anybody and everybody died of the disease. But the Hippocratics believed that people who lisp are particularly liable to diarrhoea, and the author of *Epidemics I* evidently felt that any one of the characteristics he so carefully enumerated— age, skin colour and texture, hair colour and texture, eye colour, voice, temper, lifestyle—might prove to have prognostic significance. For these were either indicators of the internal composition of the body or (in the case of lifestyle) influences upon it.

Thus survival or death depended on interpreting a range of signs that the same text lists as follows:

> First we must consider the nature of man in general and of each individual and the characteristics of each disease. Then we must con- sider the patient, what food is given to him and who gives it—for this may make it easier for him to take or more difficult—the conditions of climate or locality both in general and in particular, the patient's customs, mode of life, pursuits and age. Then we must consider his speech, his mannerisms, his silences, his thoughts, his habits of speech or wakefulness and his dreams, their nature and time. Next we must note if he plucks his hair, scratches, or weeps. We must observe his paroxysms, his stools, urine, sputum and vomit. We look for any change in the state of the malady, how often such changes occur and their nature, and the particular changes which induce death or a crisis. Observe, too, sweat- ing, shivering, chill, cough, sneezing, hiccough, the kind of breathing, belching, wind, whether silent or noisy, hemorrhages and hemorrhoids. We must determine the significance of all these signs.

At the heart of this enterprise was *prognosis*. Doctors knew they would be blamed if patients died unless they took the precaution of announcing in advance that treatment was hopeless. They needed to know, therefore, 'for a patient with fever to grind his teeth, unless this be a habit continued from childhood, is a sign of madness and death. If this occurs during delirium, it is a sign that the disease has already taken a fatal turn.' The preoccupation with prognosis reflected an imperfect recognition of the limits of the doctor's capacity to intervene. Galen (AD 131–201) said prognosis properly included the subdisciplines of diagnosis (identifying the patient's present condition) and a form of mnemonics (identifying the patient's past conditions); but both were subsidiary to prognosis. Skill at prognosis, in traditional Hippocratic/Galenic medicine, in fact served as a substitute for skill in therapy. Hippocratic doctors were able to reliably identify the signs of imminent death. But they could do nothing to delay its arrival.

The Hippocratics were good at setting bones and lancing boils, at hands-on manipulation. But none of their therapies directed at internal conditions worked. Moreover, for all their careful observation and all their prognostic skills, their basic model of the internal workings of the body was a decisive obstacle to their going on to develop any effective remedies. Yet their basic repertoire of remedies continued to be the staple of medical practice until the mid-nineteenth century. The story of Hippocratic medicine after the first Hippocratics is one of intellectual development, but therapeutic continuity.

Because in later centuries all doctors came to agree with each other, because a unified medical profession eventually came to exercise an effective monopoly over treatment, it is easy to assume that from the beginning doctors thought alike. But in fact, within these shared assumptions, there was considerable disagreement amongst the first Hippocratics, and disagreement remained commonplace throughout the classical period. It is not until 1200 that a single body of medical doctrine established an unchallenged predominance both in Islam and in Christendom. Some early doctors, including perhaps Hippocrates himself, believed that health and disease were all a matter of *pneuma* or vital spirit. Others were particularly concerned with two fluids that they believed were pernicious in excess, phlegm, which was particularly problematic in the winter, and associated with upper respiratory tract problems, and bile, which was particularly problematic in the summer, and associated with stomach problems, and they sought to explain other diseases with reference to these fluids: epilepsy, for example, was held to be brought on by phlegm. Around the time of Hippocrates' birth a philosopher called Alcmaeon of Croton had argued that health depended on a balance or equilibrium between three sets of opposing forces—hot and cold, dry and wet, sweet and sour—while the supremacy of any one of them (the language he uses is political for his term for supremacy is *monarchia*) would cause disease.

It seems to have been Hippocrates' son-in-law, Polybus, who, in a text called *The Nature of Man*, first argued that there were four humours or fluids which needed to be brought into balance to establish health (blood, phlegm, yellow bile or choler, and black bile or melancholy), that each of these four humours tended to be predominant at a different age in life and a different season of the year, and that each represented a pair of the fundamental qualities that a philosopher called Empedocles had argued went to make up the universe: the hot and cold, the dry and wet. Thus blood was hot and wet, phlegm cold and wet, yellow bile hot and dry, black bile cold and dry. Each tended to congregate in a different organ: blood and all the other humours were manufactured in the liver; phlegm went to the brain, yellow bile to the gallbladder and black bile to the spleen. From the first it was assumed that predominance of any one humour would have psychological effects, black bile, for example, leading to melancholy.

It might be thought that there was an inevitable tension between a four-humour system and, where the fluids were concerned, a threefold therapeutic practice (bloodletting, emetics, and purgatives), and perhaps practice was more in line with an earlier system which had thought in terms of three humours—blood, bile and phlegm. Black bile was apparently a new discovery, later defined by Galen as the dregs or sediment of the blood, that which lay at the bottom if blood was allowed to stand and separate. Black bile, we may suspect, was invented to bring medicine into harmony with the cosmology of

Empedocles. But it was also believed that all four humours were to be found, in varying proportions, in the blood, and that they separated out when blood was left to stand. It was thus easy for bloodletting to come to be regarded as the sovereign remedy, far more important than emetics and purgatives.

In Galen's view 'Whatever sickens the body from internal evil has a twofold explanation, either plethora or dyspepsia.' Dyspepsia resulted from eating the wrong foods; plethora from consuming more food than one burnt up or excreted. Why, in the case of one patient, did a severe wound heal without becoming infected, while in the case of another a tiny scratch became infected, red, swollen, and potentially fatal? Because the second patient was already suffering from a plethora, an excess in the blood. Without this the scratch would have been insignificant. Bloodletting thus became a cure for almost all conditions. Celsus, for example, in the first century AD, recommended bloodletting for severe fever, paralysis, spasm, difficulty in breathing or talking, pain, rupture of internal organs, all acute (as opposed to chronic) diseases, trauma, vomiting of blood. It was still being used as a nearly universal remedy in the middle of the nineteenth century.

In the ancient world bloodletting had its opponents. The followers of Erasistratus (c.330–255 BC) thought bloodletting was dangerous, and preferred to get rid of excessive blood by fasting. But the main disputes were over where to let the blood from, for some said it should be from close to the affected organ, some from as far away as possible, and over how much to let: the leading authorities were prepared to let blood up to the point when the patient fainted. Disputes over these matters were to continue as long as the tradition of ancient medicine survived. In 1799 Benjamin Rush (one of the signatories of the Declaration of Independence) was advocating 'heroic' bloodletting, and was accused by some of killing his patient, George Washington, through his commitment to this practice. The dispute was still not over whether to let blood, but rather over how much to let and where from. A critic of excessive bloodletting still regarded moderate bleeding as the pre-eminent medical remedy in 1839, and around 1870 the naturalist Charles Waterton attributed to frequent bloodletting his success in keeping himself 'in as perfect health as a man can be'.

Through the centuries, many doctors recommended a regular regime of prophylactic bloodletting, particularly in the spring. In Philadelphia in the 1830s it was still the custom, as it would have been in a medieval monastery, for people to go en masse to the doctors to be bled each spring. Such bleeding was held to be essential for those who did not vent their excess of this humour by natural means: in the case of women, in their periods, and in men in nosebleeds, varicose veins, and haemorrhoids. These last three were seen as examples of natural self-therapy. It is obvious to us, in the twenty-first century, that a nosebleed, a bleeding vein, or a bleeding bottom needs treatment; for centuries, by contrast, these were welcomed as ways in which the body healed itself. Women who had ceased to have periods (an interruption in periods, without pregnancy, in someone of child-bearing age was regarded as extremely dangerous) and men who had no haemorrhoids had to turn to doctors for an artificial substitute.

The goal of ancient medicine was a balance of humours. An early text, *Airs, Waters, Places*, argued that different climates would tend to produce a predominance of different humours, hence different physiological types and national characters. This process was seen as complex, even contradictory. Thus Galen held that the Germans and Celts, because they lived in a cold, wet climate, had soft, white skin, while the Ethiopians and Arabs had hard, dry, and black skin. But the Germans and Celts bottled up their internal heat within themselves: 'Whatever internal heat they have has retreated, along with the blood, into the internal organs; and there the blood churns about, confined in a small space, and boils; and thus they become spirited, bold, and quick-tempered.' To achieve a healthy body and disposition you thus needed to counteract the effects of the climate and the season—in summer, and in Germany, you would want to cool your blood; in winter, and in Africa, to heat it.

Under normal circumstances our control over our bodies depended upon manipulation of what Galen called the non-naturals, contrasting them to the naturals (over which we have no control—climate, season, age, sex, etc.) and the unnaturals (those conditions that were directly associated with disease). The non-naturals were food and drink, the environment (e.g. exposure to the air), sleep and waking, exercise and rest, evacuations (including sexual), the passions and emotions. A major difference between medicine in the time of Galen and medicine six centuries earlier, in the time of Hippocrates, was that Galen was convinced that we could fundamentally control the conditions needed for health; this involved sharply downplaying the role of climate and season compared to the views expressed by the Hippocratic writers, for whom a change in the direction of the wind had been sufficient to explain an outbreak of illness—Sydenham's wish to link diseases to times and places represented a return to Hippocrates and a rejection of Galen.

Just as the humoral theory implied that certain humoral imbalances fostered certain states of mind, so it assumed that certain mental conditions (e.g. anger) had physiological consequences. Mental health and physical health were thus regarded as inseparable, indeed as strictly indistinguishable. This is particularly clear from the records of Dr Johannes Storch, who practised in the German town of Eisenach in the 1730s. These contain numerous cases of women prescribed bloodletting after a fit of anger or a fright—both, it was believed, stopped the normal flow of menstrual blood, with possibly fatal consequences. One young woman of 21 was frightened 'by a dog which barked loudly at her at the time when her menses were flowing'. The flow was interrupted and did not recover; a few months later she was suffering from 'heart-throbbing, tiredness, bad colour, strong and uncommon sweating, with a strongly itching scorbutic blister'. Within the year she was dead. The dog's bark had proved as fatal as any bite.

Galen, and all doctors after Galen, thus advocated proper diet. Galen recommended a diet designed to thin the humours, consisting of fish, fowl, barley, beans, onions, and garlic for all chronic diseases. They recommended sensible exercise. Galen abhorred gymnastics as too violent—the claim that gymnastics was the science of health and medicine the science of disease seemed to him to take no account of sports injuries—but recommended instead 'exercise with the small ball', a game of catch. They recommended the regular use of laxatives and prophylactic bloodletting. But they also recommended control of the passions, particularly anger.

Galen says:

> In my youth . . . I once saw a man in a hurry to open a door. When he could not get it to open, he began to bite the key, to kick the door, to curse the gods; his eyes went wild like those of a madman, and he was all but frothing at the mouth like a wild boar. The sight caused me to hate anger so much that I would never appear thus disfigured by it.

He had particular contempt for those who struck out at their slaves. His father

> frequently berated friends who had bruised their hands in the act of hitting servants in the teeth. He would say they deserved to suffer convulsions and to die from the inflammations they had sustained. Once I even saw a man lose his temper and strike his servant in the eye with a pencil, causing him to lose the sight of one eye. And it is related of the emperor Hadrian that he once struck one of his household staff in the eye with a pencil, causing him to lose the sight of one eye. When Hadrian realized what had happened, he summoned the servant and agreed to grant him a gift of his own request in exchange for the loss he had suffered. But the injured party was silent. Hadrian repeated his offer: that he should request anything he wished. At which the servant grew bold and said that he wanted nothing but his eye back.

In Galen's eyes such behaviour unmanned those guilty of it. His mother, temperamentally the opposite of his father (an architect), was 'so bad tempered she would sometimes bite her maids'.

This preoccupation with the passions might seem a purely autobiographical obsession of Galen's, reflecting his desire to be like his father not his mother. We could also relate it to his professional circumstances. He found himself in constant competition with doctors from different schools. He would put on public exhibitions to demonstrate the superiority of his understanding of anatomy, and accost other doctors to engage them in public disputations. In such circumstances winning involved a cool head; a display of anger or irritation could only make one look weak and inadequate. But the idea of self-control was also central to his understanding of human biology.

In many respects Galen was a Platonist: he admired the *Timaeus* and thought it evident that the human body had been designed by a divine architect. He agreed with Plato, who thought there were three principles of life in the human body, reason (located in the brain), spirit (located in the heart), and appetite (located in the liver), rejecting Aristotle's argument that all life was centred in the heart (Aristotle thought the function of the brain was to refrigerate the blood). But he was completely unpersuaded by Plato's arguments for the immortality of the soul, preferring to regard it as 'a mixture or faculty of the body', and so mortal. For later generations of Muslim and Christian medical commentators, Galen's account of the relationship between mind and body was profoundly unsettling. Not for nothing did it become a saying amongst Renaissance Christians that where there are three doctors you will find two atheists, while in the seventeenth century Thomas Browne's *Religio Medici*, the religion of a doctor, is intended as a paradox or puzzle. For Galen, unlike Plato, your body is who you are. Understanding how the body worked was thus the key, not only to physical health, but also to psychological well-being.

2

ANCIENT ANATOMY

Hippocrates and his contemporaries knew remarkably little about human anatomy, the structure of the bones aside. They made no systematic distinction between arteries and veins. They could not distinguish nerves and tendons. They did not understand that muscles contract, and they very rarely used the word for 'muscles', normally speaking of 'flesh'. This may seem surprising, as the sculptors of the fifth century BC portray heavily muscled bodies, and Greek athletes must have worked endlessly to develop their muscles. But in the language of the fifth century what was admirable about an athlete's body was that it was (as modern translations have it) 'articulated' or 'jointed'. A better translation might be to say that fifth-century Greeks admired 'definition', but they had no idea that muscles are required for definition. The contemporaries of Hippocrates not only lacked the idea of 'muscles', they also had no word for the stomach. They thought the womb wandered around the female body, not only mounting into the chest, where it might cause suffocation, but even climbing as far as the head or descending into the big toe. They had no understanding of the role of the lungs in breathing, believing air went into the brain and belly. Crucially, their knowledge of the internal organs was based on what they could see when dealing with wounded patients and what they could learn from butchered animals. It is clear they never practised dissection on the human body: respect for the bodies of the dead, even of dead enemies, was fundamental to Greek culture.

Aristotle was the first to practise dissection (and perhaps vivisection) on animals. All societies cut up animals, and not just to eat them: many societies, including the ancient Greeks, foretold the future by inspecting the insides of animals. What was new in Aristotle was his conviction that every part of the body fulfilled a function: Aristotle invented the notion that the body is made of organs (the word originally means 'tools') that are designed to serve a purpose. Aristotle believed the soul uses the body to serve its purposes, and it does so through the organs. Dissection for Aristotle was thus the study of function. He looked inside the bodies of animals to find out what each part *did*. And what he found was evidence of craftsmanship. The first detailed anatomical description is a description of the heart that is to be found in one of the pseudo-Hippocratic writings. The heart, it tells us, is 'a piece of craftsmanship', and this is the language that echoes through all later accounts of human anatomy.

The first to practise dissection on the human body was, it seems, Diocles, who was perhaps a pupil of Aristotle, and who wrote a now-lost book on anatomy. Aristotle's teaching that 'when the soul departs, what is left is no longer an animal, and that none of the parts remain what they were before, excepting in mere configuration' perhaps helped overthrow what had been a fundamental taboo against cutting up human bodies. But the major revolution in anatomical thinking took place in Alexandria as a result of the work of Herophilus and Erasistratus, who were both born around 330 BC. According to later accounts they both practised vivisection: Alexandria was a despotism in which Greeks ruled over barbarians, and they may have been permitted to experiment on convicted criminals. Herophilus, in particular, established the anatomy of the brain and its relationship to the nerves, whose role in controlling movement he recognized. He also studied the reproductive organs, identifying the ovaries and the Fallopian tubes, and rejecting the view, which was still prevalent two thousand years later, that the womb moves about the body. Herophilus's teacher, Praxagoras, introduced a systematic distinction between arteries and veins, though he assumed (as did Erasistratus) that the arteries carried air, and gave to them the name also given to the trachea. It was Praxagoras who first identified the arterial pulse: Aristotle had thought that the heart and all the blood vessels pulsed together because he was unable to distinguish arteries from veins. Herophilus later explored the possibility of using the pulse for diagnostic purposes and devised a portable timepiece to measure its speed. As for Erasistratus, it is easy to mock his belief that in the uninjured body blood is confined to the venous system, while the arteries carry air; but he did accurately identify the heart as a pump with valves, even if he took it to be a form of bellows pumping air.

What emerged from the work of Alexandrian anatomists was a major revolution in the understanding of the body and its relationship to the mind. In Homer, writing in the eighth century BC, there is no general term for body or for mind. Moreover Homer has no way to say that someone made up their mind: he talks about the gods deciding what they should do. By the time we get to Aristotle in the fifth century BC soul and body are contrasted terms, and deliberation is a capacity of the soul. Moreover, the soul acts through the body, but some actions are deliberate, and some actions (e.g. breathing) take place without thought. After Herophilus there are two systems in the body. On the one hand the brain, the nerves, and the muscles (the word now becomes of crucial importance) control voluntary movement. On the other hand the heart, the arteries, and the veins represent systems over which the mind has no control, systems of involuntary action. This involved distinguishing terms that, for the followers of Hippocrates, had been near-equivalents. For the first Hippocratics the difference between pulses, palpitations, tremors, and spasms was merely one of scale: such tremblings could be seen in any part of the body. After Herophilus, the pulse (singular now instead of plural) occurred simultaneously and involuntarily in the heart and arteries; palpitations, tremors, and spasms were now afflictions of the nervous system, involuntary twitches of a system that should be under conscious control.

The first Hippocratics had never taken the pulse of their patients, but now the pulse became a key source of information about the involuntary system, as opposed to the voluntary one. We now begin to get some sense of why the idea of self-control was so important to Galen. To be human was to be in control of those bodily activities that were voluntary; to lose control, to strike and bite, was to allow the passions to seize control, and so to become an animal rather than a human being. There was, however, a fundamental ambiguity in this way of thinking. One could treat the voluntary and involuntary systems as two aspects of the human body, as Galen did, or one could see them as reflecting a fundamental distinction between the physical and the mental, between body and soul, between the passions and reason. If one went down this alternative route, dissection, which had started as a study of function, could now be said to have confirmed a fundamental claim of Socratic philosophy: that the mind was separate from the body, that mental functions and bodily functions were different in nature. Thus the distinction between the veins and arteries on the one hand, and the nerves on the other, along with the reconceptualization of 'flesh' as 'muscles', was the physiological proof of the new philosophy. Previously not only had veins and arteries been lumped together as blood vessels but nerves and tiny arteries had not been distinguished. Now anatomy had shown that one could trace the contrasted ideas of voluntary and involuntary action through the finest details of the dissected body. How could one control those functions of the body over which one had no conscious control? It was medicine's responsibility to answer this question.

After Herophilus and Erasistratus not only vivisection but also dissection seem to have ceased. For several hundred years anatomical knowledge stood still because doctors no longer had access to bodies. One of Galen's earliest works was an edition of the *Anatomy* of Marinus, and it seems that Marinus had turned to the dissection of apes in order to learn about human anatomy. Modern scholars believe that Galen himself never had an intact human body to dissect, and that his knowledge—which was, as we shall see later, extensive—derived from both dissection and vivisection of apes.

It is easy, when reading a work such as Galen's *On Anatomical Procedures*, to be struck by the extent to which his knowledge of anatomy coincides with our own. But it is important always to remember that his understanding of biological processes is fundamentally different from ours. Consistently, Greek doctors read the outside appearance of the body, and the substances excreted from it, as a sign of what is going on inside. Take hair. The Greeks were aware that the pores of the body transpire; when the vapour leaving the body is sooty, Galen held, a deposit could build up in the pores.

were themselves symptoms of an underlying imbalance of the humours; it was therefore the patient, not the disease, that had to be treated. To work through the list of Hippocratic medicaments, as modern scholars do, looking for ones that we would take to be effective—not lettuce, for sure—is to miss the point that drugs were rarely 'specifics', directed at specific diseases (the case for such drugs was first argued by Paracelsus in the sixteenth century, using the example of mercury as a treatment for syphilis), and that our belief, for example, that bathing a wound in a liquid containing alcohol might have an anti-bacterial effect would have been incomprehensible in a world where there was no concept of infection. One of Harvey's claims for his theory of the circulation of the blood was that it at last made it possible to understand how drugs could quickly take effect throughout the body; without such a theory all drugs had to be understood as being local in their impact. Prior to Harvey, *materia medica* was first and foremost about ointments, not drugs, even when they were ingested into the body. And what these ointments could be understood to do was constrained by the humoral theory that governed their use. Between Polybus and Galen that theory had been developed and refined. For the next fourteen or fifteen hundred years doctors were more concerned to preserve and transmit this intellectual inheritance than to question or improve it.

3

THE CANON

When Celsus wrote about medicine in AD 40 he identified three main schools of medical practitioner. The 'dogmatists', the followers of Herophilus, believed we must look for hidden causes in order to explain biological processes, and therefore believed in vivisection and dissection, even if they had no opportunity to practise either. The 'methodists' had a simple mechanical account of disease as the result of particles travelling either too quickly or too slowly through the body, and believed a doctor could be trained in six months. And the 'empirics' rejected all theories of disease, insisting that we must learn from past experience which sorts of intervention are effective. A century later, Galen (who was a dogmatist) was arguing with the same groups, and if we look at early Arabic medicine, in the tenth and eleventh centuries, we find several competing traditions, all claiming to be descended from Greek antecedents.

Yet, a thousand years later, in both Arab and Christian lands, Galen had established himself as the one reliable authority on medical questions. This was perhaps because he was deeply interested in logic, and so his texts fitted well into a programme of education grounded in the Aristotelian syllogism. Moreover, Galen's understanding of the body was, unlike that of the methodists and empirics, entirely compatible with an Aristotelian preoccupation with function. There may have been important differences between Aristotle's account of human biology and Galen's, in their understanding of the function of the brain, for example, and, as we shall see, in their views on reproduction, but these were marginal compared to their overall compatibility.

So we can plausibly explain Galen's survival; but it is almost impossible now to look back to the world in which Galenic medicine faced competition, because what survive are the books of Galen, not those of his competitors; the Hippocratic texts survive in large part because Galen declared himself to be a follower of Hippocrates and wrote commentaries on key Hippocratic texts. Galen certainly intended to dominate the field of medicine, and wrote at enormous length to achieve this effect—the modern edition of Galen's works in Greek runs to ten thousand pages, and much has been lost; much too survives only in Arabic translation. This copious production and trust in the written word must certainly have helped ensure his future dominance

Knowledge of Greek medicine spread in a series of waves. The first Greek doctor to be invited to Rome was Archagathus in 291 BC, and over the next five hundred years Greek doctors became more and more frequent in the capital of the Roman empire: Galen himself made the journey to Rome. By AD 500 there was general agreement in Alexandria on the key texts by Hippocrates and Galen that should form part of every doctor's education. These texts were translated into Arabic in the ninth century, particularly by Hunayn ibn Ishaq (Johannitius, d. 873) of Baghdad. Many were then translated from Arabic into Latin by Constantine the African (d. 1087), in southern Italy, and by Gerald of Cremona in Toledo in the mid-twelfth century. It was these texts, along with translations of Arabic works, which formed the foundation of medical education in the new universities of the early thirteenth century: medical education was formalized in Montpellier by the 1220s, although the first medical degree we know of was awarded in 1268, and there was little university medical education outside Bologna, Paris and Montpellier until the mid-fourteenth century, a century which saw a flurry of translations directly from the Greek.

With the printing press there came a new search for texts: a 'complete' edition of Galen in Greek was published in 1525, and this made generally available for the first time the key text for an understanding of Galen's anatomy, *On Anatomical Procedures*, of which the first Latin translation appeared in 1531. It is very striking that Galen's best work had only been available for a few years when Vesalius claimed to be able to improve on Galen—up until 1531, it was always possible to assume that Galen indeed knew best, it was just that his best work had yet to be made available.

An abbreviated edition of Galen's *On the Use of Parts of the Body*, which includes frequent references to dissection, had long been available, and it was in the mistaken belief that he was imitating Galen, who actually dissected apes not people, that Mondino de' Luzzi in Bologna in 1315 began to teach anatomy by the public dissection of a criminal's corpse; a year later he wrote the first Latin textbook on human anatomy. Already in twelfth-century Salerno pigs had been dissected for anatomic instruction. Dissections of human cadavers to ascertain cause of death had taken place for some time before 1300; and the thirteenth-century practice of boiling up the bodies of Crusaders so that their bones could be returned to their homeland (banned by a papal bull in 1299) may have prepared the way for a new willingness to cut up the dead. The new activity of public dissection was slow to spread: the first public dissection took place in Spain in 1391, in the German territories in 1404, and it did not become standard until Vesalius established it as a central part of medical education in the mid-sixteenth century. In the eighteenth century it became normal for every student to have some experience of dissection, which led to a severe shortage of bodies and a trade in the dead known as 'body snatching'.

Meanwhile, Greek medicine, as transmitted through Arabic, continued to be the foundation of all medical education. The summary of medical knowledge in the *Canon* of Ibn Sina (known in Latin as Avicenna, d. 1037), translated into Latin in Muslim Spain by Gerald of Cremona in the 1140s, continued to be used as a textbook at Montpellier until 1650, and at some Italian universities until the eighteenth century. So important was this text that an edition in Arabic was published in the West in 1593. In 1701 the great Dutch physician Boerhaave gave his inaugural lecture 'in praise of the Hippocratic school' and as we have seen Sydenham was admired as 'the English Hippocrates'. It was the Sydenham Society that produced the major translation of Hippocrates into English in 1849. Doctors thus had a set of key texts in common from AD 500 to 1850.

Galen would consequently have had little difficulty making sense of a university education in medicine at least until the mid-seventeenth century, when new discoveries in anatomy began to come thick and fast. He would have been interested to see that his scattered comments on diagnosis from inspection of urine had been assembled to form a new discipline, uroscopy, which had taken shape in late fourth century Alexandria: among the texts translated by Constantinus Africanus was an Arabic text on the subject. And he would have been dismayed to discover that the Arabs had wedded medicine closely to astrology, and that this linkage had become part of university education in Latin Europe, so that doctors routinely took horoscopes to decide on treatment: in Valencia in 1332 it was decreed that barber surgeons must consult qualified doctors, or physicians as they had begun to be called since the early thirteenth century to reflect their university education in Aristotelian natural science, before bleeding their patients: this was to ensure that they did so only on days which were astrologically favourable. Galen himself had opposed the use of astrology (which had been imported into Graeco-Roman medicine from Babylonia). He had, on the other hand, edited with approval the Hippocratic text *Regimen*, which advocates diagnosis from a patient's dreams. To dream of a rough sea, for example, 'indicates disease of the bowels. Light and gentle laxatives should be used to effect a thorough purgation'. But, except for the interest in astrology, he would easily have recognized medicine in 1650 as a direct continuation of medicine in 200.

4
THE SENSES

Hot, cold, dry, wet seem to us simple terms, in principle susceptible to measurement. Galen was much interested in the question of whether the young were hotter and colder than the old. He believed he had trained himself to so exactly remember heat that he could compare the warmth of the same person several years apart, and he decided, after extended observation, that, as we might say, their temperature was the same. Or rather he decided something quite different, for though the temperature was the same,

> there are differences in the quality of the heat . . . that of children is more vaporous, large in quantity, and sweet to the touch; while that of people in their prime verges on the sharp, and is not gentle at all . . . [it is] small, dry, and less gentle. Neither therefore is hotter in any simple sense, but the former appears so . . .

Heat was for Galen a complex, not a simple, quality.

We should not be surprised, then, that Celsus, when he comes to discuss fever, hastens to stress that a patient should not be regarded as feverish just because he feels hot—he may have been working hard, sleeping, or he may be suffering from fear or anxiety. We can only conclude he has a fever if he not only feels hot and has a rapid pulse, but

> if also the surface of the skin is dry in patches, if both the forehead feels hot, and it feels hot deep under the heart, if the breath streams out of the nostrils with burning heat, if there is a change of colour whether to unusual redness or to pallor, if the eyes are heavy and either very dry or somewhat moist, if sweat, when there is any, comes in patches, if the pulse is irregular . . .

Consequently it will not do just to touch the patient's skin. The doctor must face him 'in a good light, so that he may note all the signs from his face as he lies in bed'. The thermometer was invented by Sanctorius Sanctorius, a friend of Galileo's, in the seventeenth century; but we can be sure that if Celsus had had a thermometer he would not have felt that it alone could provide proof of a fever. Indeed it is striking that the thermometer only became a standard clinical tool with the death of Hippocratic medicine, spreading from Berlin (where Ludwig Traube introduced it around 1850) to New York (1865) and Leeds (1867). In 1791 Jean-Charles-Marguerite-Guillaume de Grimaud was still arguing that the patient's temperature as measured by a thermometer was of little interest. Nothing could substitute for the physician's hand. 'The doctor must apply himself, above all, to distinguishing in feverish heat qualities that may be perceived only by a highly practised touch, and which elude whatever means physics may offer.' Thus feverish heat is acrid and irritating; it gives the same impression as 'smoke in the eyes'.

What would seem to us one of the simplest of all substances, water, was almost infinitely complex for Hippocratic doctors, who recognized, perfectly sensibly, that it varied immensely from place to place: the title of *Airs, Waters, Places* identifies it as one of the three crucial environmental variables. 'No two sorts of waters can be alike,' asserts this author, 'but some will be sweet, some salt and astringent and some from warm springs.' Water from marshes and lakes will be 'warm, thick and of an unpleasant smell in summer' and 'productive of biliousness. In winter it will be cold, icy and muddied by melting snow and ice' and 'productive of phlegm and hoarseness'. There is also water from rock springs ('hard, heating in its effect, difficult to pass and causes constipation'); water from high ground ('cool in summer and warm in winter', and, if it flows towards the north-east, 'sparkling, sweet-smelling and light'); water which is salty and hard (good for the phlegmatic); rain water ('very sweet, very light, and also very fine and sparkling' but unfortunately it also 'quickly becomes rotten on standing'); water from snow and ice ('always harmful [for] in the process of freezing the lightest and finest part has been dried up and lost'); while water from large rivers or from lakes into which many streams flow is particularly likely to produce a sediment of sand or slime and to cause stone, gravel in the kidneys, strangury, pain in the loins and rupture.

Before drinking water, then, you needed to know exactly where it had come from. To live in a town which was forced to take water from a lake would be to condemn oneself to a potentially endless cycle of colds and diarrhoea. The Romans may have used aqueducts to deliver adequate supplies of fairly clean water to large cities, but water did not begin to be treated to make it safe to drink until after Pasteur's germ theory of disease. Before then water was sometimes filtered, or even chemically treated, to prevent it from smelling foul, but not to kill germs. So we can easily agree with the Hippocratics that water was a major cause of disease, but not with their explanation that it might not only be too salt, too sweet, or too astringent, too hard or too soft, but also too hot or cold, too light or heavy.

Five hundred years after *Airs, Water, Places*, Celsus sums up this analysis of water with what appears to be admirable simplicity by classifying water in terms of degrees of heaviness, except for the fact that he defines heavy waters as those which have the most nourishment and are hardest to digest.

> Rain water is the lightest, then spring water, next water from a river, then from a well, after that from snow or ice; heavier still is water from a lake, the heaviest from a marsh . . . by weighing the lightness of water becomes evident, and of water of equal weight, that is the better which most quickly heats or cools, also in which pulse is most quickly cooked.

Heaviness, here, both is and is not a matter of weight.

When it came to more complicated foods even more numerous factors had to be taken into account. Thus, according to an early fourteenth-century manuscript produced for use in Bohemia, but itself a translation of an eleventh-century Arabic original, *The Almanac of Health*, roosters are dry and hot; not surprisingly then they are recommended for people of a frigid complexion, in old age, in winter, and in northern regions, such as Bohemia. But could we have predicted that the best roosters are those that crow temperately, or that rooster meat can cause irritation of the stomach that can be avoided if the birds are tired out before they are slaughtered, presumably by chasing them around the farmyard? Clearly an old, cold man suffering through a northern winter could not just order rooster for dinner: his cook needed to have known the rooster in life and in death. And a doctor who advised his patient to eat rooster, and found him the next day suffering from indigestion, could easily dismiss the problem, saying the rooster selected had been too vocal or insufficiently exercised.

The multiplication of relevant factors meant that the Hippocratic doctor could always explain away failure. When Taddeo Alderotti (d. 1295) was called out to treat the count of Arezzo, who had been taken ill, he found the patient improving, and left him in the care of his students. The next day he returned to find him at the point of death. How could his prognosis have been so seriously mistaken? He searched around until he discovered that he had not noticed an open window, at which point he was satisfied that the cold night air provided an adequate explanation.

If doctors were just like astrologers (in fact they were normally one and the same people) in having available numerous tactics for explaining away failure, medicine was rather different from astrology in that it appeared to give patients control over their own fate. Since health lay in a balance of humours, and such a balance could be obtained through a correct regimen (a correct management of the non-naturals) everyone ought to be able to achieve health. Just as we might think that someone with a hangover has brought it upon themself, so ancient medicine (at least after the Alexandrian revolution in anatomy) implied that someone who was ill was in some degree responsible for their own condition. Although we believe that people who choose to live high-pressure lives may bring on heart attacks, we rarely blame people for getting cancer or arthritis; ancient medicine, by contrast, implied that all diseases reflected deficiencies in lifestyle. In some respects this empowered patients. Are you an old man who wants to make love to a young woman? Then eat the right food first—pigeon breasts are particularly recommended. (You will find a more detailed menu in the Roman author Terence's play *Clizia*; in the Renaissance Machiavelli translated the play, and the advice would have seemed entirely up to date.) Are you a scholar, living a sedentary life, and so prone to the scholar's disease, melancholy? Then you need exercise: a sea voyage perhaps (travelling in a coach or a boat was, like rocking, taken to be a form of exercise), or regular horse-riding. When Montaigne wrote an essay 'On Coaches' he expected you to understand that coach journeys can have a therapeutic function. In the eighteenth century Adam Smith, the founder of economics, prescribed horse-riding to himself to counteract the deleterious consequences of too much book-reading, and it must be said this still seems a sensible prescription.

As a result the burden of responsibility often lay heavy upon the patient. 'Physicians come to a case in full health of body and mind' says the author of the Hippocratic *Science of Medicine*, taking it for granted that no one would hire a doctor who was not able to ensure his own health. Patients, by contrast,

> are full of disease and starved of nourishment; they prefer an immediate alleviation of pain to a remedy that will return them to health. Although they have no wish to die, they have not the courage to be patient. [*Note the automatic and unthinking reference to the three topics with which medicine concerns itself: the alleviation of pain, the restoration of health, the deferral of death.*] Such is their condition when they receive the physician's order. Which then is more likely? That they will carry out the doctor's orders or do something else? Is it not more likely that they will disobey their doctors rather than that the doctors . . . will prescribe the wrong remedies. There can be no doubt that the patients are likely to be unable to obey and, by their disobedience, bring about their own deaths.

Medicine defined itself as a science by transferring responsibility for failure, firmly and remorselessly, from doctor to patient.

One last example may serve to illustrate what it was like to live in a world, not of quantities, but of qualities. As we have seen, Praxagoras was the first to understand the pulse as an involuntary movement of heart and arteries, and his pupil Herophilus was the first to use it as a diagnostic tool, classifying pulses by magnitude, strength, rate, and rhythm. It was only for the third of these measures that his timepiece would have been useful. Galen went further. He wrote at enormous length on the pulse: a thousand printed pages survive. In *The Pulse for*

Beginners he explains that arteries have three dimensions—length, depth, breadth. In other words, in order to understand the pulse he immediately thinks of the anatomy of the body as exposed by dissection. The pulse itself must be considered in terms of its strength, hardness, speed, interval, regularity, and rhythm. Thus a pulse could in theory be large, long, broad, deep, vigorous, soft, quick, frequent, even, regular or, at the opposite extreme, small, short, narrow, shallow, faint, hard, slow, sparse, uneven, and irregular. In anger, he tells us, the pulse is deep, large, vigorous, quick, and frequent; in pleuritis quick, frequent, hard, and, consequently, you can be deceived into thinking it is vigorous (for remember, strength and hardness are different dimensions of the pulse). Galen devised evocative terms to identify particular types of pulse. Thus the 'anting' pulse is extremely faint, frequent, and small. Such a pulse appears quick but is not: speed and frequency again are different dimensions.

To train oneself to identify different types of waters by their taste, or different types of pulse (and Galen thought the pulse the most valuable of all diagnostic tools), was to acquire a level of connoisseurship that in our society we would expect to find only in a wine merchant or a restaurant critic. Galen himself says that his knowledge of pulses is not something that can adequately be expressed in words. It involved a distinctive and elaborate expertise of the touch. But was this expertise real? Galen spent years trying to decide whether he could 'feel' the contraction of the artery as well as its expansion. For later generations the question of just what one could and could not feel was to be a matter of unending dispute, a dispute which parallelled the unending dispute over how much one should bleed and where from. In Galen's own day the empiricists insisted that there was an enormous gap between the faint fluttering sensation at the end of one's fingertips and a general theoretical claim about the heart and the arteries. In the eighteenth century we find frequent expressions of scepticism. Duchemin de l'Etang in 1768, after months of study, decided that the study of the pulse was treacherous: 'I began to suspect that there might be a bit of enthusiasm and imagination behind the whole matter.' William Heberden in 1772 advised the Royal College of Physicians to attend only to 'the frequency or quickness of the pulse', which is the only quality that is identical in all parts of the body. He protested that 'the minute distinctions of the several pulses exist chiefly in the imagination of the makers'. One might think there was something peculiarly modern about Heberden's desire to make the pulse something one could measure, but Herophilus had measured pulse beats. In doing so he had had to measure smaller units of time than anyone had previously conceived of: the beat of an infant's pulse was, he thought, the irreducible minimum unit in the measurement of time.

By the early seventeenth century Sanctorius Sanctorius (he of the thermometer) had a pendulum machine to measure the pulse rate, and John Floyer had developed a suitable watch by 1707. In 1733 the first accurate measurements of blood pressure were taken (although measuring the blood pressure involved killing the animal; the first proper measurement in humans dates to 1828, and was on a limb about to be amputated). By the mid-nineteenth century machines that measured both pulse rate and the difference between systolic and diastolic pressure (the sphygmograph) were in widespread use, while the modern method of measuring blood pressure dates to 1896. But eighteenth-century expressions of scepticism about the value of the pulse, and early attempts to reduce the pulse to measurable quantities, were in part a response to attempts to restore to the pulse an importance that few after Galen had been prepared to give it. For centuries doctors had preferred to diagnose from samples of urine rather than from subtle distinctions in the pulse. It was easy to produce a colour chart that showed how to interpret different shades of urine; impossible to portray or quantify the subtle sensations that Galen had claimed to feel in his fingertips.

Elaborate forms of sensory expertise have not entirely disappeared from medicine. Doctors are still trained to identify a wide range of bumps and murmurs through their stethoscopes (Laennec was so proud of his invention that he claimed one could learn much more from a stethoscope than by feeling the pulse); but in our world there are very few forms of scientific knowledge that cannot be expressed in pictures or numbers, but depend instead on taste, touch, sound, or smell. As late as early 1930s, however, the young Karl Stern in

Frankfurt was still being trained in a medicine that depended on sensory expertise:

> There was . . . an entire world of touch which we had never perceived before. In feeling differences of radial pulse you could train yourself to feel dozens of different waves with their characteristic peaks, blunt and sharp, steep and slanting, and the corresponding valleys. There were so many ways in which the margin of the liver came up towards your palpating finger. There were extraordinary varieties of smell. There was not just pallor, but there seemed to be hundreds of hues of yellow and gray.

Hippocratic doctors thought the body's excretions were the best indication of what was happening within, and bodily excretions often assault the senses. Not surprisingly, Hippocratic doctors had little choice but to use all their senses. *Prognosis* tells us that, for example, 'the best kind of pus is that which is white, smooth, homogeneous and least foul smelling. That of the opposite sort is the worst.' (Only after Lister did doctors come to think of all pus as bad.) Ancient Greek doctors listened to the lungs by pressing an ear to the patient's chest: modern doctors still hear through their stethoscopes the sound 'like leather' that characterizes certain lung diseases and was first described by the early Hippocratics. They tasted ear wax: if it was sweet death was imminent, if bitter recovery could be expected. Galen rejected the claim that the heart was a muscle, not only on the grounds that one could not control its beat, but also on the grounds that if one cooked and ate a heart it tasted nothing like flesh. The four humours (blood, phlegm, yellow and black bile) each had to be examined with care. According to Avicenna, phlegm could be sweet, salty, acid, watery, mucilaginous. According to Maurus of Salerno in the twelfth century, blood could be viscous, hot or cold, slippery, foamy, fast or slow to coagulate. You had to observe the layers into which it separated, and once it had separated the solids should be washed and their texture felt—slippery blood was a sign of leprosy. When Celsus inspected urine he noted its colour, whether it was thick or thin, its smell, and its texture (was it slimy?): black, thick, malodorous urine was a harbinger of death.

Sight was particularly important. We have seen Celsus stress that the doctor must have a good view of his patient. Every doctor was trained to look out for the change in facial appearance that marked the imminence of death: the nose becoming pointed, the temples sunken, the eyes hollowed, the ears cold and flaccid with the tips drooping slightly, the skin of the forehead hard and tight. You could see death approaching. But touch was also fundamental. The first Hippocratics always palpated the hypochondrium, literally the parts under the cartilage, that is, the sides of the abdomen under the ribs. In a memorial statue of a doctor from the second century AD we can see him reaching out to his patient to touch him here, where he is evidently swollen. The Hippocratic text *Prognosis* discusses at length what you could expect to learn by feeling a patient here, and concludes: 'In brief, then, painful hard large swellings [of the hypochondrium] mean danger of a speedy death; soft, painless swellings which pit on pressure mean protracted illness.' A hypochondriac was originally someone with something wrong with their hypochondrium; it was only in the nineteenth century, when the hypochondrium ceased to be of medical interest, that the term was freed to refer to someone who was mistaken in their belief that they had something wrong with them (there had long been a term in French for such people: they were *malades imaginaires*). An early Hippocratic, if he could have watched Karl Stern, in the 1930s, as he felt for the margin of the liver with his finger, would have understood him to be palpating the hypochondrium.

Since the humours were classified in terms of hot and cold, dry and wet, then these were all directly experienced by touch. Galen thought long and hard about whether our experience of hot and cold, dry and wet was objective or subjective. His conclusion was that it was objective because human beings had been designed to be, when in health, at the objective midpoint between the four extremes: healthy humans were neither hot nor cold, neither dry nor wet when compared to other humans; but they were also so when compared to the universe as a whole. Moreover in the body it was crucially the skin, and of the skin it was above all the skin of the palm of the hand which had reliable sensation: the hands 'were designed to be the instrument of assessment of all perceptible objects', created as 'the

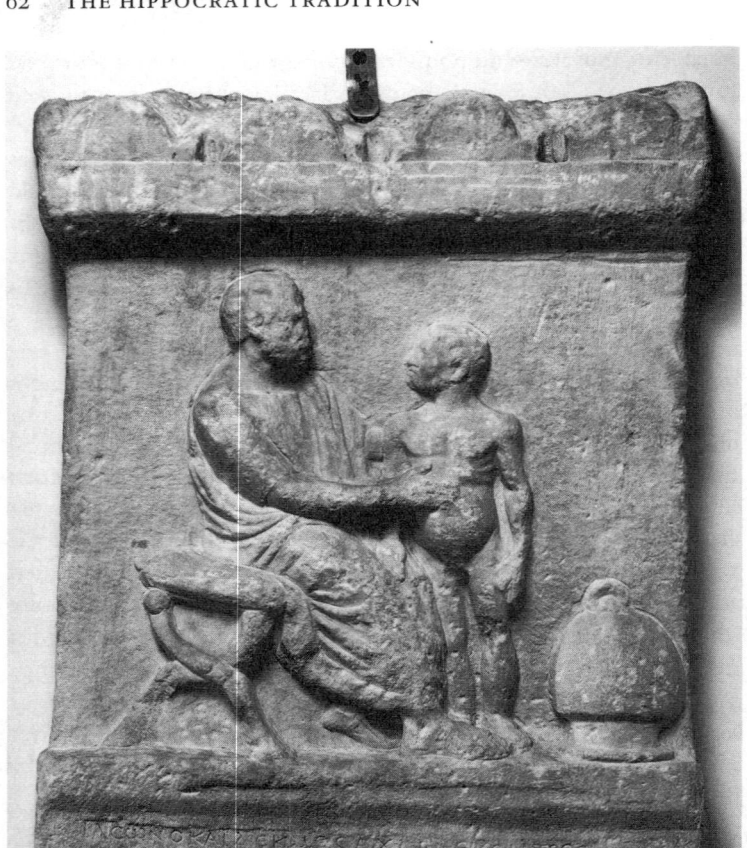

6. The tombstone of Jason, an Athenian doctor of the second century AD. On the right is a cupping vessel, not to scale.

organ of touch suited to the most intelligent of all animals. It therefore had to be equidistant from all extremes.' Skin provides 'the
standard or yardstick against which to examine all other parts of the
animal'. To function as the yardstick, however, the doctor himself had
to be in perfect health, his own body a proper balance of the
humours, his skin neither cold nor clammy, neither feverish nor dry.
For Galen medicine was above all a tactile science.

In medieval Europe this hands-on idea of medicine came under
immense pressure. From the early thirteenth century surgery was
normally separated from medicine (as it had briefly been at the very
beginning—in the original Hippocratic Oath doctors promise not to
use a knife): this was not entirely true in Italy, where the occasional
university degree in surgery was bestowed; but throughout Northern
Europe medicine and surgery soon became different professions, and
surgery was normally taught outside the universities, though it too
was taught on the basis of Greek and Arabic texts. Underlying this
was a conviction that the educated should not engage in manual
activity. To define surgery, as Guglielmo da Saliecto did, as 'a science
teaching how to operate manually on the flesh, nerves, and bones of
man' was to mark its liminal status as requiring both education and
manual labour. As surgery and medicine became for the first time
separate professions, the very act of touching seemed an activity for a
surgeon not a doctor. When Vita and Letizia da Villa Casale took
their young son, who was suffering from a hernia, to the doctor he
told them to go to a surgeon for 'touching and cutting'.

What made possible this retreat from touch, this novel situation
where doctors were no longer in touch with their patients, was a new
conviction that diagnosis was possible on the basis of a urine sample
alone. The urine bottle was now the symbol of the doctor, where
once it had been the cupping vessel or the hand on the hypochondrium. In the new Latin Kingdom of Jerusalem in 1245, the law
provided that if a patient died under medical treatment, the doctor
should be whipped around the streets, holding a urine bottle in his
hand, and then hanged. Sick people regularly sent samples of their
urine to the doctor, making a bedside visit unnecessary. William
of England wrote a text entitled *If one cannot Inspect the Urine*. The

answer was not to visit the patient, but to cast his horoscope. In seventeenth-century England, there were plenty of medical practitioners who were happy to diagnose on the basis of a urine sample and an astrological chart. A sample of urine had become an epitome of the patient's whole body, a genuine substitute for it. When doctors did visit their patients, taking their pulse represented a form of polite touching: even Galen had recommended taking the pulse at the wrist as that did not require the patient to undress. When called to advise the emperor he hesitated even to touch his wrist until he was urged to do so.

One of the factors at work in this retreat by doctors from physical contact with the bodies of their patients was certainly a fear of contact between the sexes. In the earliest Hippocratic texts, doctors conduct vaginal examinations themselves; soon though they expect women to conduct them on their behalf. The Athenian Agnodice was, according to legend, one of Herophilus' pupils. Distressed by the anguish of women who would rather die than be examined by a man, she cross-dressed in order to study medicine so that she would be able to treat women. In an Arab manuscript an illustration of the use of a vaginal speculum shows a woman conducting the examination, and there were apparently Arab female physicians, and female specialists in opthalmology and surgery. Nevertheless, in both East and West, there were men who also practised gynaecology and obstetrics, and when in 1322 a female unlicensed healer in France claimed she should be allowed to practise medicine as she would not endanger female modesty her plea was rejected—the first woman to qualify as a doctor in modern times was Elizabeth Blackwell in America in 1849. Through the Middle Ages, it seems, male doctors were prepared, on occasion, to palpate the hypochondria of their female patients, but in the early modern period such contact was increasingly regarded as inappropriate. Greater even than the new prohibition against touching was the prohibition against seeing. In 1603 Edward Jorden described a physician and a surgeon treating a tumour on a young maiden's back. The physician 'modestly put his hands under her clothes' to feel it; the surgeon wanted to 'take up her clothes, and to see it bare', a suggestion at which she was 'greatly offended'.

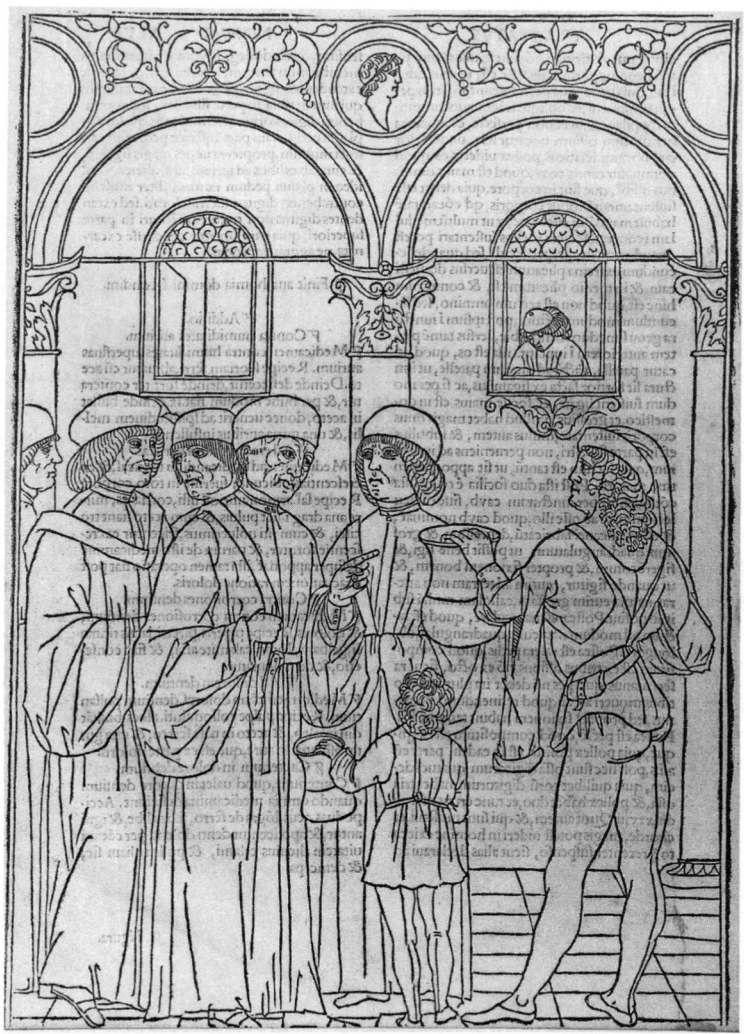

7. A doctor inspecting urine in a urine bottle – the patient is not present. This image first appears in 1493, and is reproduced from Johannes de Ketham, *Fasciculus Mediciniae* (Venice, 1522).

It is only in the light of medicine's retreat from direct contact with the body that we can understand the medical practice of Johannes Storch (b. 1681), the eighteenth-century German doctor we met in Chapter 1, who published extensively on women's diseases. In the majority of his cases, Storch never met his patient, relying on letters and messages, or the reports and requests of intermediaries. Even when a patient came to Storch, or Storch went to see a patient, Barbara Duden tells us,

> in most instances he did not touch her for the purposes of examination. Here too he acted on the basis of what the patient said and what he could find out in further conversation. The importance of words and the public nature of the complaint stand in sharp contrast to the unimportance of a medical examination and what one can almost call a taboo against touching . . .

When women occasionally show him (never at his request) parts of their bodies (a lump on a breast, a hernia, a lump on her right side) they do so 'with great embarrassment', 'with great modesty and embarrassment', 'bashful[ly]'. Of one he records, 'since she was expected to die, she agreed to have her naked body looked at and touched'. In this society (and many other early modern societies may have been similar) only the dead were exposed to the hand and the eye. Only in the nineteenth century did the living become once more exposed to the doctor's touch, and even then great caution had to be used; as we have seen, the original function of Laennec's stethoscope was to overcome the fact that he could not possibly put his ear to a woman's chest. Family doctors, visiting patients in their homes in the United States in the 1890s, usually contented themselves with feeling the pulse and inspecting the tongue.

CONCLUSION TO PART I:
THE PLACEBO EFFECT

Put simply, the fundamental puzzle about medicine from the fifth century BC until the end of the nineteenth century is that doctors found patients who were prepared to pay for treatment that was at best ineffectual, and usually deleterious. Throughout this period surgery, particularly abdominal surgery, was commonly fatal, while the most common therapies were bloodletting, purging, and emetics, all of which weakened patients. Advances in knowledge, such as the discovery of the circulation of the blood, had no pay-off in terms of advances in therapy, so that we might say that all the progress was in human biology, none of it in medicine. At the end of the seventeenth century, Charles Perrault, in his *Parallèle des anciens et des modernes*, felt quite safe in having the spokesperson for the ancients dismiss all modern anatomical discoveries as irrelevant to treatment. Looking back to the beginning of the century, Arthur Hertzler, a Kansas doctor, wrote in 1938, 'I can scarcely think of a single disease that the doctors actually cured during those early years ... The possible exceptions were malaria and the itch. Doctors knew how to relieve suffering, set bones, sew up cuts and open boils on small boys.' In 1905 Joseph Matthews, a past-president of the American Medical Association, felt that the only drugs physicians really needed were laxatives and emetics.

But the fact that there was no progress—far too little to have any systematic impact on life expectancy—and the fact that medical intervention did more harm than good, does not mean that doctors did not cure patients. Modern studies of the placebo effect show that it is a mistake to think that there are some therapies that are effective and others which though ineffective work on those who respond to the placebo effect. Even effective medicine works partly by mobilizing the body's own resources, by invoking the placebo effect: one estimate is that a third of the good done by modern medicine is attributable to the placebo effect.

When patients believe that a therapy will work, their belief is capable of rendering it surprisingly efficacious; when doctors believe a therapy will work their confidence is consistently transferred to the patient. There are all sorts of studies that show this in practice. Thus if a new and better drug comes out, the drug it replaces begins to perform consistently less well in tests, merely because doctors have lost confidence in it. If doctors administer efficacious drugs believing them to be placebos, then their effectiveness is less than if they administer them believing them to be efficacious. If you change the size or the colour of a pill, or the number of times a day it is administered, you alter its effectiveness. Patients who faithfully follow their doctors' instructions do better than those who do not, even if the pills they are being instructed to take are inert.

It is important though to stress that if Hippocratic medicine benefited its patients by mobilizing the placebo effect, Hippocratic therapies were not in themselves placebos. Placebos are inert substances, and new drugs are regularly tested against placebos in blind clinical trials—a drug has to outperform a placebo before it is regarded as having any therapeutic effect. But Hippocratic remedies were far from inert. Bloodletting, purging, and emetics acted powerfully and, in so far as they acted on the body, they were bad for patients. In so far as they acted on the mind they may have been good for patients, but we can be confident that if one tested Hippocratic remedies against placebos the placebos would outperform the Hippocratic remedies: doing worse than a placebo is, if you like, a technical definition of what I am calling 'bad medicine' or 'doing harm'. By this definition, which I think is the appropriate one, you are doing harm even if your patient is more likely to recover as a result of receiving your treatment than if he had received no treatment at all, providing your treatment is less beneficial than a placebo. The doctor Foucault tells us about, who abandoned Hippocratic remedies and gave all his patients quinine, was giving them a better therapy, not because quinine is effective, but because he was coming closer to giving a true placebo.

Homeopathy, founded by Samuel Hahnemann, who published his *Handbook of Rational Healing* in 1810, is regarded by conventional modern doctors as working by mobilizing the placebo effect, and homeopathic remedies are held to be inert substances. What homeopathy can do for you is thus a good indication of what a placebo can do for you, and, on the definition I am proposing homeopathy does neither good nor harm, though it is perfectly reasonable that it should be available (as it increasingly is) on the National Health Service, since it performs much better than no treatment at all. Homeopathy, we can be sure, would have outperformed Hippocratic medicine in a trial. It follows, then, that for the first hundred years or so homeopathy was superior to conventional medicine; it is only for the last hundred years that conventional medicine has had a strong claim to be superior to homeopathy. We can be confident then that medicine has always been better for patients than no treatment at all, but until the late nineteenth century the benefit of treatment usually derived solely from the fact that doctors and patients believed it would be beneficial, and consequently it was.

We can also be clear that the type of benefits that medicine was capable of offering, until the last century, and leaving aside some simple surgical procedures and a very few other treatments, was effectively restricted to what the body is capable of doing for itself. Thus if a patient takes a placebo believing it to be a pain-killer they are likely to experience a reduction in pain, and this reduction is not just in the mind: the body produces endorphins, which reduce the pain. In this way the placebo can mimic the working of opiates. But the body is incapable of producing a substance comparable to aspirin (introduced in 1899), so that even if you take a placebo believing it to be aspirin, the body will never successfully mimic the action of aspirin; your pain relief will still come from the production of endorphins. Before 1865, as after, doctors were able to marshal all the resources of the placebo effect, and it is a safe general rule, to which there were, as Hertzler acknowledged, very few and very limited exceptions (setting bones, reducing dislocations, operating for bladder stones and cataracts, and, in later periods, taking opium for pain relief, quinine for malaria, digitalis for dropsy, mercury for syphilis, orange and lemon juice for scurvy), that this is all that medicine could do. For more than two thousand years medicine effectively stood still, despite all the progress in human biology, and a doctor in ancient Rome would have done you just about as much good as a doctor in early nineteenth-century London, Paris, or New York.

But if modern medicine is effective and Hippocratic medicine was not, it follows that the very idea that there is continuity between the two is profoundly misleading. The same institutions may educate doctors in the twenty-first century as in the thirteenth (you can still get medical degrees at Bologna, Paris, Montpellier); many of the same words may be used to describe diseases; but modern medicine is no more a development of ancient medicine than modern astronomy is a development of medieval astrology. The two are fundamentally different. At the very beginning of the twentieth century, on the other hand, the medical care that could be offered by doctors such as Hertzler and Matthews was still essentially Hippocratic. Bleeding had been largely abandoned (though it continues to be used even at present for two fairly rare conditions, hereditary haemochromatosis, a disease of excessive iron storage in the body, and polycythemia, a complication of severe lung disease), for it made no sense for those diseases that were now thought of as infections; and humoral theory had given way to modern physiology; but laxatives and emetics were still the doctor's basic remedies. Twenty years earlier, and the standard therapies were even closer to those of Hippocrates: in 1878 Émile Bertin, in his article on bleeding in the *Dictionnaire encyclopédique des sciences médicales*, is still recommending bloodletting for a wide range of conditions, and supporting his argument by appeals to Galen and Thomas Sydenham, 'the English Hippocrates'. This was still bad medicine. Bertin's patients would have been better advised to go to a homeopath.

II. REVOLUTION POSTPONED

5

VESALIUS AND DISSECTION

Ten years ago my daughter went to medical school. In her first week, they introduced her to a corpse, and asked her to start cutting it up. As it happens, she is a vegetarian, and if they had asked her to cut up a raw leg of lamb I am not sure she could have coped. There were six on her dissecting table, one of whom dropped out. My daughter is now a psychiatrist: raw flesh is not for her.

Since the nineteenth century, dissection has been a rite of passage, the beginning of a medical education. If you cannot face cutting up the dead, how will you be able to slice into the living? For centuries (until computer imaging made it possible to move around and through a body) dissection was the only reliable way to learn anatomy, and the dead body the only place you could afford to make mistakes. In this tradition of medical education, the great hero is Vesalius (1514–64), who is regarded as the founder of modern medicine. The beginning of modern medicine can then be dated to a day in 1536 when Vesalius, walking outside the city walls of Louvain, came across the body of an executed criminal chained to a gibbet. Only the bones remained, 'held together by the ligaments alone'. Vesalius at once made off with the arms and legs, but came back that night (defying the curfew) to climb the gibbet, smash the chain and carry off the trunk. Out of these parts he constructed his first skeleton —boiling them up secretly, and then pretending that he had brought them with him from Paris. 'I was burning with so great a desire to possess those bones,' he wrote seven years later, 'that I did not hesitate to snatch in the middle of the night that which I so desired.' Vesalius had no name for his desire, and I can think of none either. The love of knowledge certainly formed part of it. So did a burning desire to imitate Galen, who describes coming across a rather similar skeleton in his *On Anatomical Procedures*, a work which had only recently been rediscovered, and a translation of which had been published by Vesalius's teacher, Guinter of Andernach, in 1531. But so too did a delight in doing what no one else dared do, what was forbidden. At night restless spirits walk, and Vesalius was one of them.

In Northern Europe dissection was a relative rarity, and Vesalius went on to conduct the first dissection in Louvain for eighteen years. Vesalius complained that his own education at the University of Paris had been so pathetic that, despite being a medical student who had practised only on the bodies of animals, he had had to take over from the instructor during the dissection of a human being in order to show how it ought to be done. In Italy, however, dissections had been routine for over two hundred years. In 1315 Mondino de' Luzzi, at the University of Bologna, conducted the first comprehensive dissection of a human corpse for over a thousand years, perhaps even since Herophilus and Erasistratus, and the next year he published a manual on the subject. Mondino believed himself to be following in the footsteps of Galen, although there is no conclusive evidence that Galen ever actually dissected human beings.

Mondino established a new norm for medical education in Italy (where the distinction between medicine and surgery was less sharp than in Northern Europe): doctors were expected, as part of their university education, to be present at dissections. Dissections were carried out in the winter months and the bodies used were those of recently executed criminals. No more than one or two dissections were normally conducted in a year, and the audience consisted of a small group of twenty or so. As these dissections became routine, they were brought within a conventional academic framework, that of the lecture. The professor read from a textbook, usually that of Mondino, while his assistant, frequently a practising surgeon, carried out the dissection. The real object of study was the book; the body was only there to illustrate what was being described in the book. Such academic dissection was quite separate from the occasional opening up of a body to establish the cause of death, the post mortem, a process which goes back before 1315 and has a continuous history thereafter.

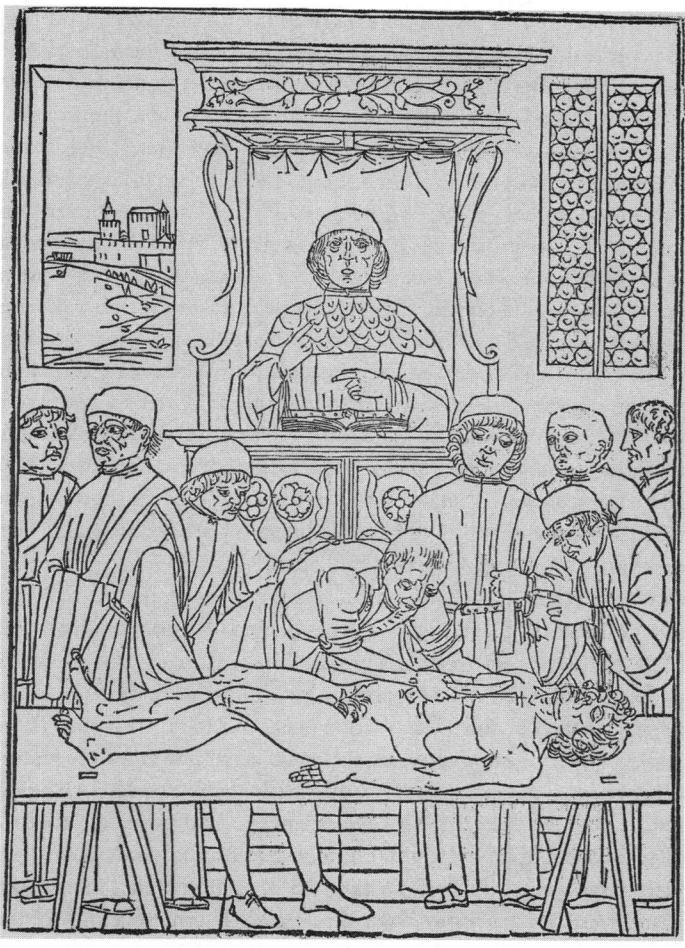

8. Anatomy Lesson, from Johannes de Ketham, *Fasciculus Mediciniae* (Venice, 1522). This illustration stands at the beginning of an edition of Mondino's *Anothomia*. In the first two editions of this collection the image is slightly different – the lecturer has no book in front of him, and is presumably intended to be Mondino himself. This reworked image first appears in 1495, and shows a lecturer reading from Mondino's text – it thus shows how anatomy was taught prior to Vesalius.

With Vesalius and his immediate predecessors (in Italy, from 1490 or so) everything changes. Dissections become much more frequent— in 1522 Jacopo Berengario da Carpi (c.1460–c.1530) claimed to have dissected hundreds of bodies. The result was a crisis in the supply of bodies. Dissections also became immensely popular. Tiered seating would be erected in a church or a square so that a very large audience could get a good view—audiences of five hundred were not unknown. The frontispiece of Vesalius's great work, the *De Humani Corporis Fabrica* or *The Construction of the Human Body* (1543), shows the crowds gathered to watch 'an anatomy' (as a dissection was called by contemporary Englishmen). Moreover such audiences consisted not just of doctors and medical students, but of philosophers, theologians, gentlemen and their servants, though, if Vesalius's frontispiece is to be trusted, there were no women amongst them. Attending a dissection was now a fashionable entertainment. By the early seventeenth century special anatomical theatres were being built in Italy and Holland for the public performance of dissections (and there were women in the audience in Holland).

Above all, the focus of dissection was now not on the book but the body: Vesalius used no book, but displayed the parts of the body himself. In the preface to the *Fabrica* he laid great stress on the need to step down from the *cathedra*, the pulpit or great chair from which professors lectured, and work with one's own hands, and the *Fabrica* contains a portrait of Vesalius dissecting an arm. The anatomy lecturer was now expected to lecture from what Vesalius called the book of nature (thus indirectly acknowledging the traditional authority of books), and this involved, quite literally, getting his hands dirty.

Why was there such public interest in anatomy in the sixteenth century? Vesalius was proud to be doing exactly what Galen had done —Galen had not trusted his slaves to prepare bodies (in his case, the bodies of apes), but had worked on them with his own hands, and had conducted dissections in public. The new anatomy fitted in with a much larger enterprise of recovering the culture of classical Rome, an enterprise that embraced literature, philosophy, and art. Vesalius, though, was convinced (quite possibly correctly) that Galen had dissected only apes, dogs, pigs, and other animals, not humans. This was

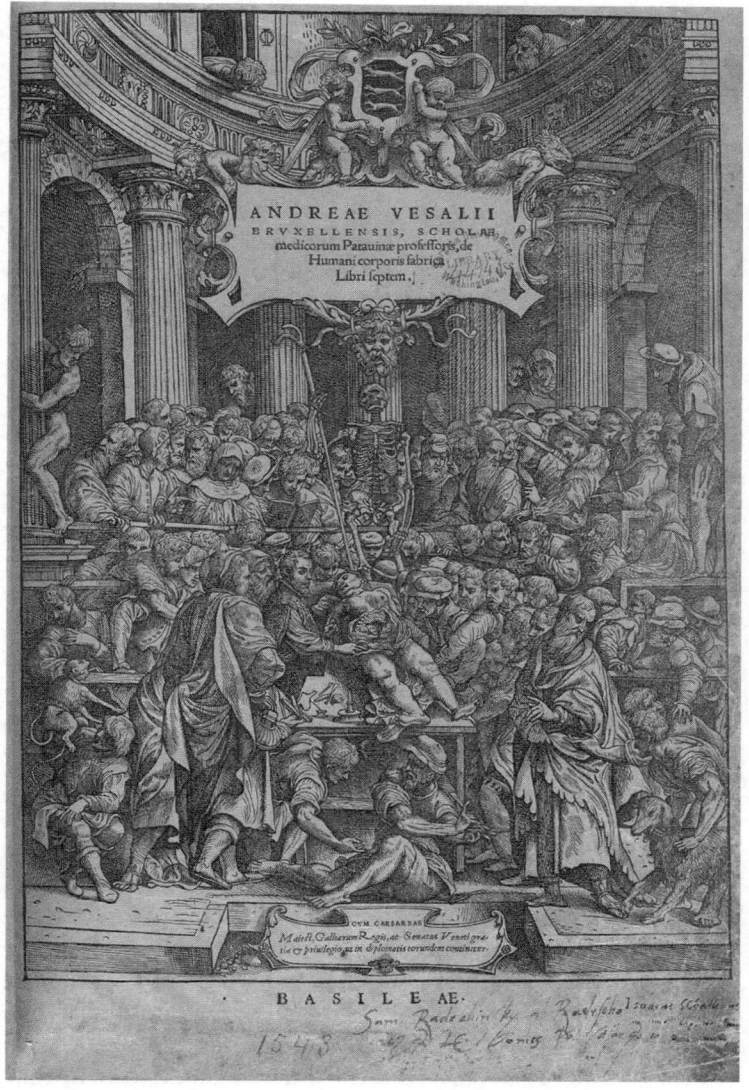

9. The titlepage to the 1st edition of Vesalius's *De Humani Corporis Fabrica*.

the only feasible explanation for his numerous mistakes: in the *Fabrica* Vesalius set out to demonstrate more than three hundred of them. At his public dissections he may well have compared dogs and monkeys with humans (both a monkey and a rather strange-looking dog appear in the frontispiece) so that people could see for themselves the source of Galen's misconceptions, but such animals were probably primarily to hand so that they could be vivisected. Anatomy thus represented new knowledge in a world where the assumption had long been that there could be no progress beyond the achievements of the ancients.

Anatomy was seen as being of central importance. It was man's knowledge of himself, through which the anatomist learnt about his own body. But at the same time man was a microcosm, a little universe, an epitome of the macrocosm or larger universe, so that all knowledge was to be found reflected and summarized in him. And man had, the Bible said, been made in the image of God, so the study of anatomy was also the study of the divine. Moreover anatomy gave onlookers the opportunity to meditate on death and the transience of life, a theme both philosophical and religious. Finally, the Renaissance did not see minds and bodies as distinct in the way that we (since Descartes) do: hair colour, for example, reflected the balance of the humours, and this determined the psychology of the individual. To study someone's body was also to study their mind. All this served to give the messy and disturbing task of cutting up bodies an extraordinary dignity.

Renaissance art had already trained people to look at the body in a new way, and from the beginning the great artists of the Renaissance had practised anatomy. Donatello (1386–1466) attended anatomical dissections (he illustrates one in a bronze, 'The Heart of the Miser') and made a bronze sculpture of the skeleton of a horse; Antonio Pollaiuolo (1432–98) 'removed the skin from many corpses in order to see the anatomy underneath'. To portray weight, balance, movement, tension, and strength the artist had to have a direct knowledge of the structure of the bones and the shape of the muscles. In 1435 Alberti advised anyone painting a human figure to imagine the bones beneath the skin and to build up from them the muscles and the surface appearance, and there is a sketch by Raphael in which he can be seen doing exactly that. The great Leonardo (1452–1519) was so interested in the structure of the human body that he planned a book on human anatomy, perhaps to be written in conjunction with a famous Florentine doctor of the day, Marcantonio della Torre. A generation later, the artists crowded round Vesalius at dissections.

On such occasions the artist and the anatomist had more in common than just an interest in bodies. At the same time that the anatomist was getting down from his podium to get his hands dirty, the artist, who had always been considered of low social class because he worked with his hands, was laying claim to a new social status, a right to mix with intellectuals and nobles. Both had an investment in dignifying manual dexterity. The anatomist was demonstrating his newfound knowledge, but the human body was interesting partly because artists had trained the public to look at it with an anatomist's eye. The anatomists and the artists, by giving manual work a new status, made possible the scientific revolution, which itself depended on the educated learning from artisans and doing things for themselves with their own hands. The anatomy theatre is the first laboratory, the cadaver the first experimental apparatus. Galileo, Boyle, and Newton followed in the footsteps of Leonardo and Vesalius, and the crowds who gathered to watch Vesalius were giving their support to the first modern scientific enterprise.

Without three technical developments Vesalius could never have accomplished what he did: the printing press using movable type; the woodcut; and perspective representation. In order to claim that he knew more than Galen had done, Vesalius had to direct his audience to reliable editions of Galen. He himself edited, for the great Giunta edition of Galen's *Opera Omnia* that appeared in 1541–2 and included many new translations from the best Greek manuscripts, the key anatomical text of Galen, the one that had inspired his own bone-stealing in 1536. An anatomist like Mondino, in the fourteenth century, could not read the full range of Galen's writings, or be sure that the copies he had were reliable (even Vesalius complained that he could not get sight of crucial Greek manuscripts that he needed to check the accuracy of the Latin translations). By 1542 any educated person with access to a decent library could trace the full range of Galen's views on any topic, and could be confident that the texts at his disposal were generally accurate. He could now claim to be sure of what Galen thought and consequently to be in a position to judge whether he was wrong or right. The printing press and the new scholarly editions that it made possible were fundamental to Vesalius's enterprise of surpassing Galen.

In addition, before the printing press medical books had had either no illustrations or only very rudimentary ones. Manuscripts were copied by hand and so only the crudest of illustrations could be employed. With anything complicated the quality was bound to degenerate as one copy was made from another. With the printing press came a new emphasis on illustration; woodcuts and (even better) copper plates could be employed to provide complex and detailed information. Leonardo saw clearly the possibilities that this opened up. Beside one of his anatomical drawings of a heart he wrote:

> O writer what words of yours could describe this whole organism as perfectly as this drawing does? Because you have no true knowledge of it you write confusedly, and convey little understanding of the true form of things . . . How could you describe this heart in words without filling a whole book? And the more minutely you try to write of it the more you confuse the mind of the listener.

Vesalius invented the process of labelling parts of illustrations with letters keyed to an accompanying text, so that readers could turn back and forth from text to illustration using each as a commentary on the other.

Vesalius was also able to draw on the great discovery of Renaissance art, perspectival representation, to produce images that created the illusion of being three-dimensional, without which it would have been impossible to represent the interrelationship of the different parts of the human body. Raised in Brussels and Louvain, educated in Paris, by 1537 Vesalius was teaching in Padua, and to illustrate his great work, the *Fabric of the Human Body*, he turned to the nearby city of Venice, to the artists in Titian's studio. The first scientific drawings employed the skills of the most highly trained artists of the day.

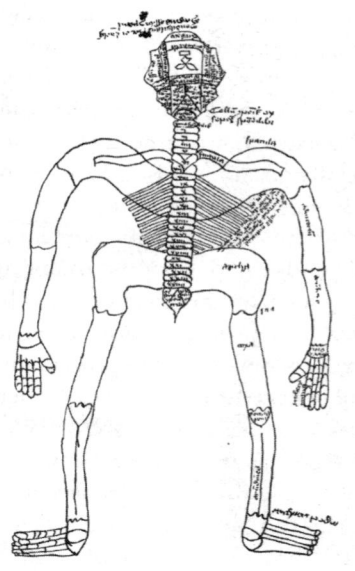 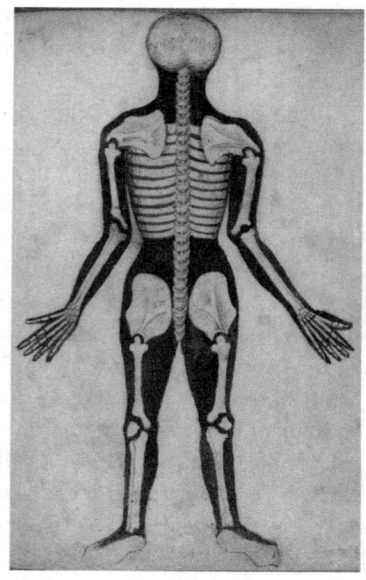

10 AND 11. These two medieval illustrations of skeletons, one from the fourteenth and one from the mid-fifteenth centuries, give an indication of the very varying quality of the illustrations accompanying medieval medical manuscripts – but even the finer of the two, an exceptionally detailed image for a medieval manuscript, falls far short of the standard of accuracy established by Vesalius.

Vesalius was the first to bring together anatomy, art, and the printing press. In principle, Leonardo could have beaten him to it; but the enterprise would have been impossible before 1500, when a lavishly illustrated book would have been hopelessly expensive (the first anatomical drawing made from direct observation had appeared in print as recently as 1493), and eccentric before 1531, for up until then the task of catching up with the knowledge of the ancient Romans was still incomplete. Before Vesalius, the most important work to pioneer anatomical illustration was Berengario da Carpi's *Commentaria* of 1521; Vesalius published his first illustrated medical text, the *Tabulae Anatomicae* in 1538, in collaboration with an artist, Joannes Stephanus of Calcar: he must have begun work on the *Tabulae* almost immediately on arrival in Padua. He was clearly determined to waste no time.

Illustration, of the quality pioneered in the *Fabrica*, enabled the anatomist to make manifest exactly what it was that he thought he had seen. His successors could compare both his words and his plates with what they found on the dissecting table, and if there was a discrepancy they could be certain that they had found something new. Leonardo carried out a number of dissections, and in his drawings we can trace the development of his anatomical understanding. At first he held all sorts of mythical beliefs derived from ancient authors: for example, that there was a duct connecting the penis to the brain, so that semen contained not only matter from the testicles, but spirit from the brain. The great English anatomist, Thomas Willis, was still looking for such a duct in the 1660s. As time passed, Leonardo made ever more exact observations of the human body, although occasionally it is clear from his drawings that he has more experience of dissecting cows than humans, so that bovine features appear in his illustrations of human anatomy! Still, his new knowledge, confined to his private notebooks, had no impact on his contemporaries. Vesalius's discoveries, by contrast, were a public record of the extent (and the limits) of his knowledge.

In the *Fabrica* Vesalius set out to illustrate the human body logically, which meant ignoring the sequence of an actual dissection. A dissection started with the abdomen, which was where putrefaction began first, and then proceeded to remove the skin, and work down through the layers of the flesh, ending with the bare bones. As a result the normal name for a skeleton in sixteenth-century English was 'an anatomy', since a skeleton was the end product of the anatomical enterprise. But Vesalius begins the *Fabrica* with the bones and they, at the end of the first book, are then assembled into a series of three elegant skeletons, viewed from front, side, and rear. He then works from the surface of the body inwards, and only finally does he turn to the abdomen. One can see at once the pedagogical advantages of such an approach, but it was also a symbolic choice on Vesalius's part: the skeleton represented the beginning of his own career as an anatomist.

Only having introduced you to the skeleton does he begin to work with the whole body.

The skeleton was Vesalius's trademark, and it became the trademark of the new anatomy. Hippocrates may have given a statue representing a skeleton to the temple of Asclepius. Galen had stressed the importance of trying to find a body where the flesh had rotted away and all the bones were in place, though there is no evidence that he ever went on, as Vesalius did, to assemble a skeleton by tying the bones together with thread and wire. There are images of skeletons on late Roman tombs and drinking cups, reminders of the shortness of life; and in the later Middle Ages there are often images of death as an emaciated creature with the bones showing through, or even as a mere skeleton. And Donatello's bronze horse's skeleton shows how natural it was for any Renaissance artist to think in terms of skeletons. There was nothing new, then, about the idea of a skeleton. Vesalius however turned the articulated skeleton into a central pedagogical aid: he had one hanging by the body being dissected as he lectured and cut, and, in imitation of him, generations of anatomists furnished every anatomy theatre with its skeleton.

Vesalius could use skeletons as pedagogic aids because he had a new method for producing them. He implies he is following the example of Galen, but the reference he gives to Galen is false, and perhaps deliberately misleading. He tells us, in the opening pages of the *Fabrica*, that his predecessors had put bodies in coffins, covered them in quick lime, and then, after a few days, cut holes in the sides of the coffins and put them in a stream. After a while, the coffins were removed from the running water and opened; the flesh had washed away, leaving the bones, still tied together by ligaments. But the dark ligaments concealed much of what needed to be seen.

Vesalius's method was very different. In his kitchen, he boiled up a large vat of water. He carved up a body, removing as much flesh as possible, and carefully putting aside loose pieces of cartilage, including the cartilage in the tip of the nose and the eyelids. He then boiled up the body until it fell apart, pouring off the fat and straining the liquid so that nothing was lost. He was left with beautiful clean bones that could be wired together to create an almost perfect representation of

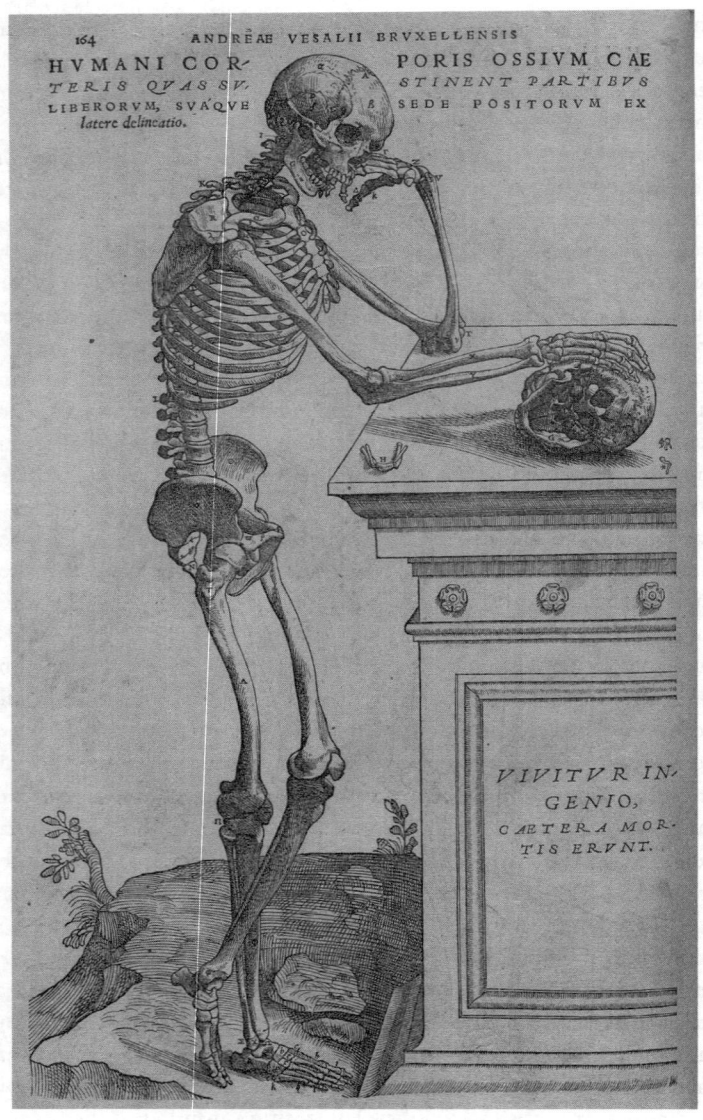

12. The lateral view of the skeleton from the *De Fabrica* of 1543.

the 'living' skeleton. Those little bits of cartilage which could not be reattached (the tip of the nose, the stiffening to the eyelid, the ears) he strung together on a necklace to decorate his teaching aid, which was then made portable by being mounted on a folding stand and encased in a box—one of Vesalius's skeletons survives to this day in Basle.

There is something profoundly alarming about the story of how to make a skeleton: Vesalius is boiling bones as if he was making beef stock; he is chopping up bodies in his own kitchen as if he were about to eat them. By beginning with bones, and with his recipe for producing skeletons, Vesalius was inevitably reminding his readers that there was something shocking about dissection. As already noted, a papal bull of 1299 had specifically forbidden the boiling up of bodies (a method used for the bones of Crusaders), and Mondino had acknowledged that there were some bones in the skull that could only properly be exposed by boiling them up: these, Mondino said, he was accustomed (a slippery word) to leave alone, in order to avoid committing a sin. Readers of Vesalius naturally concentrate on the large and elaborate scientific illustrations; but each book and then each chapter begins with an illustrated initial letter—a larger letter for the first letter of each book, a smaller one for the first letter of every chapter after the first. Naturally the first letter of the preface is a large initial V, illustrated by a picture of an anatomist cutting into a body positioned so that it seems strangely alive. The first letter of book I, facing the portrait of Vesalius himself, shows putti (naked children) boiling up bones in a kitchen to make a skeleton. The innocence of the putti contrasts sharply with the cooking of human beings. This, as much as the portrait of himself, is Vesalius's chosen self-representation.

It is sometimes said that the very act of looking inside the body was disturbing. This is certainly wrong, as in Italy it was normal to embalm bodies to help preserve them between death and the funeral. Italian funerals were 'open casket' events; no body that had been dissected could be buried in the normal way. But worse still, no body that had been turned into a skeleton could be buried at all. At the very heart of the new practice of dissection, where it ended in the production of a skeleton, was a truly shocking act: the denial of burial to the dead. Theologically speaking, one did not need to be buried in order to be resurrected to eternal life: Vesalius's skeletons, bones in a box, with the flesh torn away and boiled off, were in no worse a position as far as resurrection was concerned than fishermen drowned at sea, and Italian cemeteries contained ossuaries where old bones were collected when plots were reused for fresh burials. Still, the burying of the dead was a fundamental gesture of respect, and if the remains of the dissected sometimes ended up in a tomb, they often ended up on display.

Vesalius was engaged in a strangely contradictory activity. On the one hand he employed the finest artists to turn his cadavers into aesthetic objects. He carefully posed his dead bodies so that they could be represented as though still alive. He had them illustrated in landscapes, as if walking about. When he came to illustrate the viscera, where it was clearly impossible to make a corpse look alive with its guts hanging out, he created the illusion that an antique statue was being opened up to discover flesh-and-blood organs within. But then, he provides an illustration to show just how his bodies were posed: a corpse held up by a rope, hanging from a pulley, bits of flesh dangling from the bones. When he dissects the brain, he allows you to see (after the idealized anonymity of the 'muscle men') the moustache and facial characteristics of the corpse: his friends would be able to recognize him. And he provides an illustration of the lower torso, with legs splayed and dangling penis, which makes it look like a hunk of meat on a butcher's slab. At one moment he is a magician, beautifying death; at the next he is telling you it was only a trick, and showing you how terrible the dead body can be.

We find the same contradiction in the text. At one moment Vesalius is writing of anatomy as a divine calling, at another he is boiling human bodies in a vat. It is Vesalius who tells us that he obtained the first body he worked on by pulling it down off a gibbet and carrying it home in pieces under cover of darkness; Vesalius who tells us that his students stole the unburied body of a woman who had recently died, and quickly flayed it so that those who knew her would not recognize her; Vesalius who tells us that one of the bodies he dissected was that of a recently buried prostitute famous for her

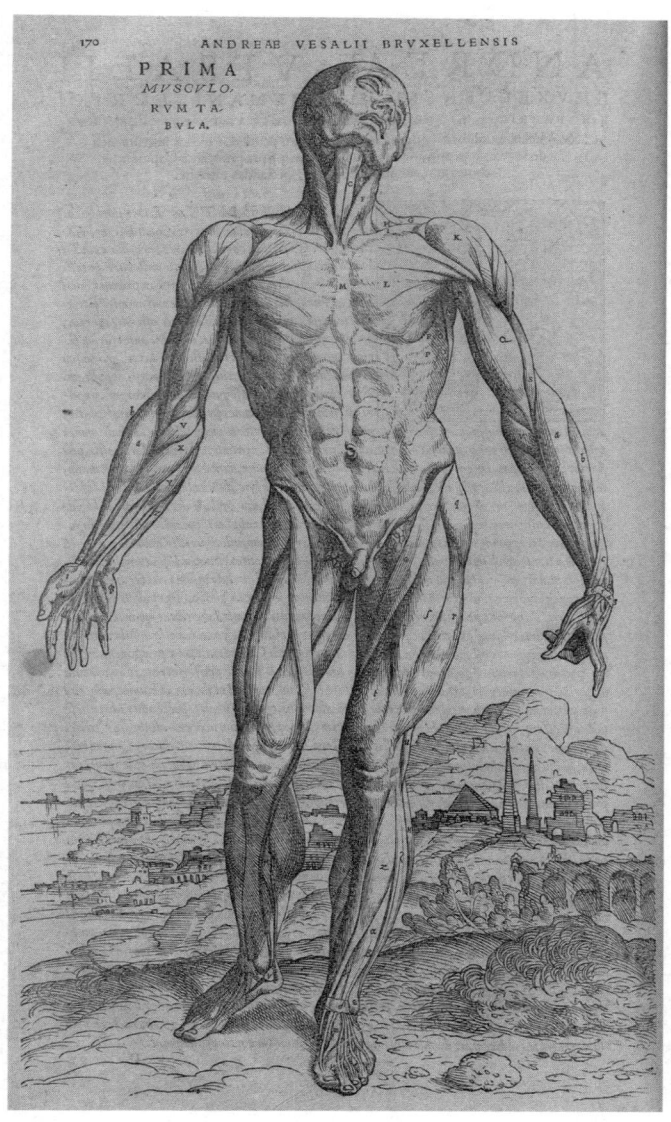

13. The first illustration of the muscles from the 1543 *De Fabrica*.

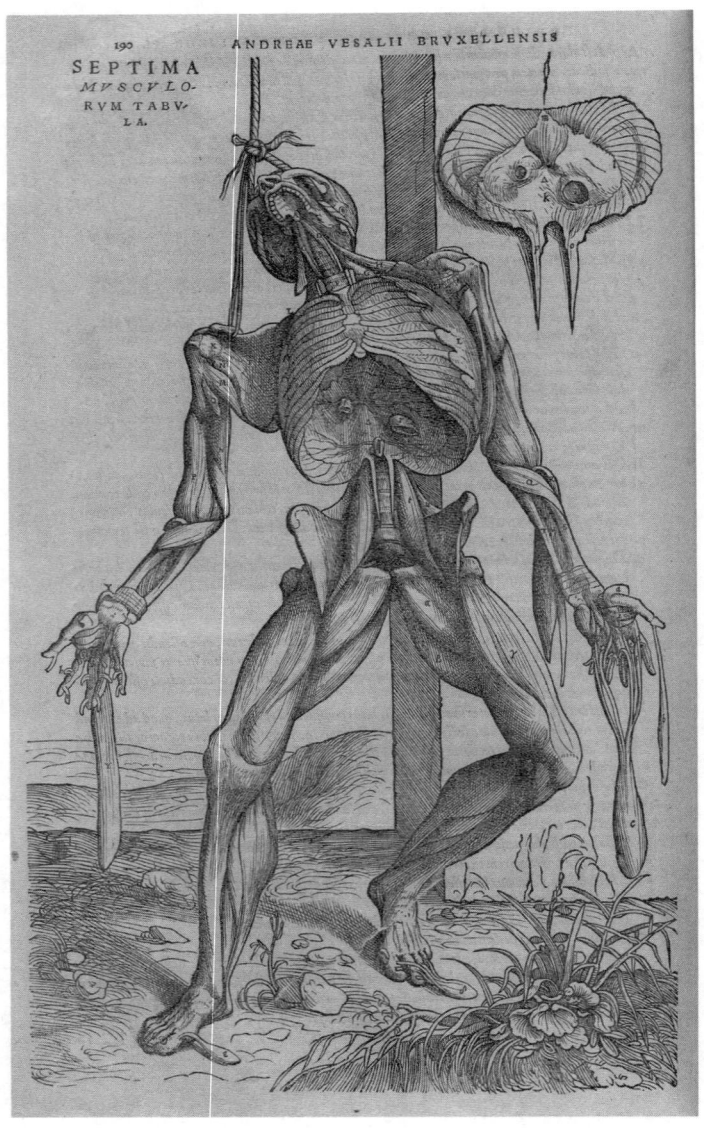

14. The seventh illustration of the muscles from the 1543 *De Fabrica*.

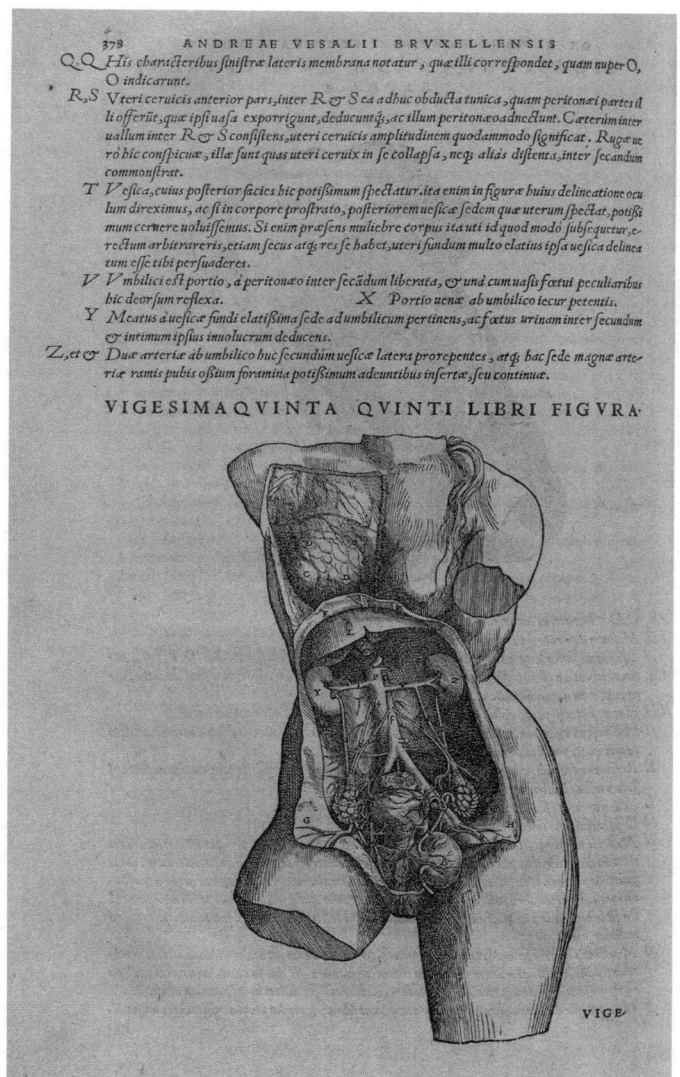

15. Third illustration of the anatomy of the torso from the *De Fabrica*: this is one of a series of images that turn the body into an antique statue.

beauty, her body stolen from the cemetery; Vesalius who tells us that his students had keys made so that they could get easy access to bones and bodies in the cemeteries. (The large initial letter 'I' which opens book VII shows putti robbing a grave.) Vesalius repeatedly tells us, in short, that he obtains bodies by stealing them and makes it absolutely clear that much of this activity is criminal: in the case of the flayed woman, her relatives went straight to a judge to protest the theft of her corpse. In 1497, the anatomist Alessandro Benedetti had claimed the law allowed the dissection of 'unknown and ignoble bodies', those of foreigners and criminals, who had no one to protect their honour, but in Venice at least the law was tightened up in 1550 to put an end to tomb robbing by anatomists, and many of the stories with which Vesalius had regaled his readers disappeared from the revised edition of the *Fabrica* in 1555.

A tiny detail in the text illustrates Vesalius's obsession with the transgressive. Once an initial letter had been designed it was reused whenever the same letter occurred: thus the large initial V that stands at the head of the preface also stands at the head of book V. But there are two small initial 'L's—the standard initial 'L' shows a body being removed from the gallows; but at the point in his text where he discusses the anatomy of the arse, Vesalius has an initial 'L' which shows a putto shitting. This is, quite straightforwardly, a dirty joke; but what Vesalius is doing here is shitting on his own book.

Vesalius was not the only one to tell stories against himself: Leonardo joked about having the quartered bodies of human beings lying around his studio, as if it was a butcher's shop. It is worth remembering that in Renaissance Europe, butchers, like executioners, were always social pariahs, forced to live on the outskirts of town, and unable to marry the daughters of other tradesmen. One artist, the sculptor Silvio Cosini, as if in a Renaissance *Silence of the Lambs*, even made a T-shirt for himself out of the skin of a dissected body: scolded by a friar, he gave his shirt a decent burial. The main legitimate source of bodies was the scaffold (remember the initial 'L' with its body being removed from the gallows), but bodies that had been executed were inevitably badly damaged. Not surprisingly, anatomists were eager to cut out the middleman; the great anatomist Fallopio (the

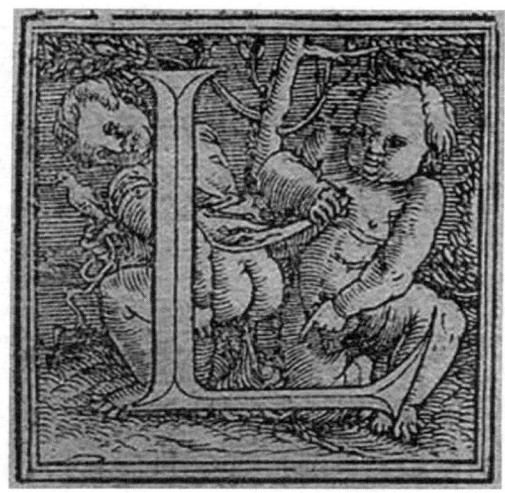

16. This initial letter 'L', which appears once in the 1543 edition of *De Fabrica*, does not appear in later editions.

discoverer of the Fallopian tubes) was given a live criminal by the ruler of Tuscany; the arrangement was mutually beneficial, for the condemned man was killed by opiates, a merciful death which left the body intact. The search for fresh corpses could also bring anatomists perilously close to human vivisection: Vesalius writes of removing the still pulsing heart of someone 'killed' in an accident.

Anatomy was an inherently transgressive activity that only slowly became respectable; for his publisher Vesalius chose not a Venetian press, but Oporinus of Basle, who had a reputation for publishing heretics (including Castellio and Servetus). Vesalius constantly emphasized both anatomy's potential for respectability and its transgressive character. One could argue that his own texts imply a subtext: that Vesalius confesses to tomb robbing and cooking up human bodies because he is himself horrified by what he does. Katharine Park has written of Vesalius's 'candid pride' in his tomb-robbing exploits, but on the contrary his behaviour suggests someone deeply conflicted. As soon as he had seen the *Fabrica* through the press he gave up lecturing on anatomy to become a doctor to the emperor; and he destroyed a number of unpublished works. He died on the island of Zante, returning from a pilgrimage to Jerusalem: according to a story we owe to the great Renaissance surgeon Ambroise Paré, he had fled Spain for the Holy Land when the body of a young girl that he was dissecting had turned out to be still alive.

Johannes Metellus tells us that on his return his ship had been caught in storms and had been at sea for forty days; those on board had not expected the voyage to be anything like as lengthy. 'Several [of the passengers] became sick, partly through lack of biscuit and partly through lack of water, and Vesalius's mind was so disturbed by the casting of the dead into the sea that he fell ill, first through anxiety and then through fear, and asked that if he should die he might not, like the others, become food for the fish.' You might think that being eaten by fish is no worse than being eaten by worms; but there is an important difference. Human beings do not eat worms but they do eat fish. To be eaten by fish is to enter the human food chain; it is cannibalism at one remove. And it was always the spectre of cannibalism that overshadowed the anatomist's art.

Fortunately for Vesalius he did not die until very shortly after reaching land, and was given a decent burial, so that, according to Pietro Bizzari, his body 'might not remain as food and nourishment for wild beasts'. 'May God preserve us from such a fate', wrote the early sixteenth-century anatomist Alessandro Benedetti after describing an anatomy. Vesalius, terrified of being eaten by fishes, would surely have been equally dismayed at the thought of being chopped up, boiled, and turned into a skeleton; to have one's body stolen by medical students was every bit as awful as being eaten by wild beasts. Concealed behind Vesalius's bravado is a genuine alarm at what he had done; we find no trace of this horror in the greatest pupil of the Paduan anatomists, William Harvey, who carried out post-mortem dissections on both his father and his brother.

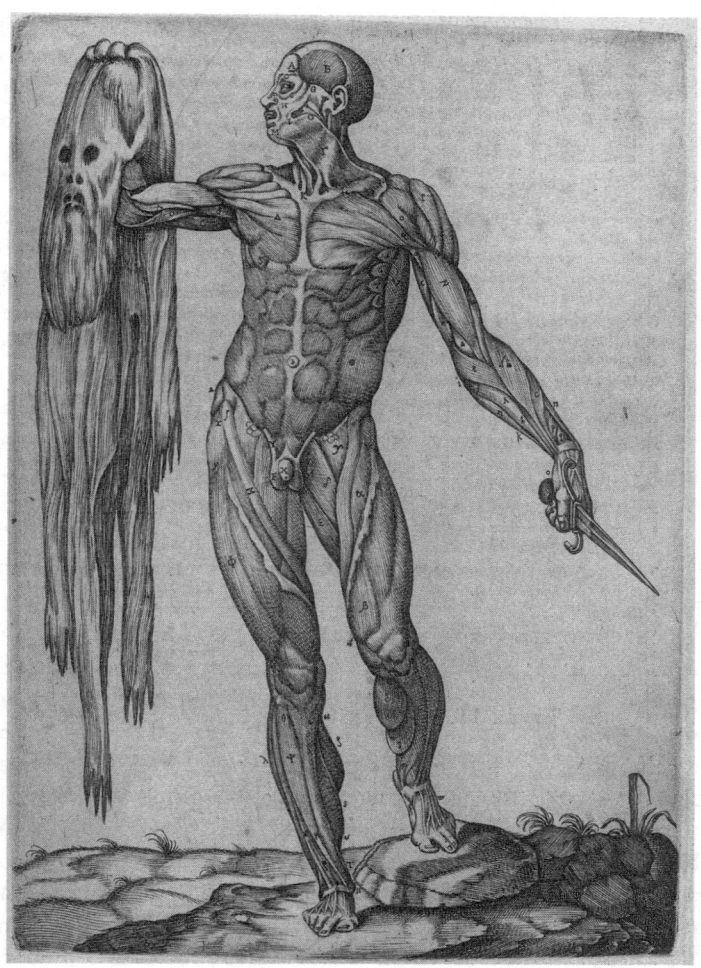

17. Most early anatomy texts (strangely, with the exception of Vesalius's *De Fabrica*) seek to make the reader forget what an actual dissection would be like by having the posed figures participate in displaying parts of themselves. In this illustration from Juan Valverde de Amusco's *Anatomia del corpo humano* (1560) an *écorché* or flayed figure holds up his own skin for your inspection.

6

HARVEY AND VIVISECTION

In 1628 William Harvey, who had received his medical education in Padua (1600-2), where the tradition of Vesalius was still very much alive, published *Exercitatio Anatomica de Motu Cordis et Sanguinis in Animalibus*—an anatomical exercise on the movement of the heart and blood in animals. *De Motu Cordis* is often regarded as the founding text of modern medical science: it is certainly the first text to set out to show that Galen was wrong on a fundamental question of biology. In order to understand its importance we need to look first at Galen's account of the movement of the blood, and then at Harvey's.

As far as Galen was concerned there were two quite separate systems involving blood in the body. The veins carried blood enriched by food through the body from the liver. This blood was dark in colour, and the tubes it ran through had thin, soft walls (the sole exception being what Galen called the arterial vein, running from the heart to the lungs, which carried dark blood but had the walls of an artery). The arteries carried blood mixed with air through the body from the heart. This blood was bright red in colour, and the tubes it ran through had thick, relatively hard walls (the sole exception being what Galen called the venous artery, running from the lungs to the heart, which carried bright red blood but had the walls of a vein). In the arteries blood washed back and forth, as in a tidal river, carrying life-giving air in one direction, and soot and other waste products in the opposite direction. So too in the veins blood moved both away from the liver (carrying nourishment) and towards it (to be replenished). In the arteries, the blood was moved by the pulsation of the arteries themselves. Galen believed that blood was manufactured in the liver, and consumed in the arteries. Thus there needed to be a slow seepage between the two separate systems, and this took place through the wall, the *septum*, between the right ventricle and the left ventricle, where small pores permitted the transfer of blood from one to the other.

Harvey replaced this account of two separate blood systems, venous and arterial, by what is still the standard modern account according to which the blood flows through two 'circular' systems: first, from the right ventricle to the left atrium, by way of the lungs; then from the left ventricle to the right atrium, travelling out through the arteries and back through the veins; a process endlessly repeated. What drove the blood through this double system were the contractions of the right and left ventricles, and the pulse in the arteries was simply the wave of blood expelled from the heart; the arteries themselves were entirely passive. On Harvey's account the arterial vein was really an artery because it carried blood under pressure from the heartbeat (even though the blood was venous in colour), while the venous artery was really a vein because it carried blood back to the heart (even though the blood was arterial in colour).

It is important to see that there were losses as well as gains in the substitution of Harvey's account for Galen's. Harvey could not account for the difference in appearance of venous and arterial blood: Joseph Priestley did not discover oxygen until 1775, so Harvey had no way of understanding that the function of the lungs was to oxygenate the blood; he could only argue that the difference between venous and arterial blood was superficial, for if the two were left to stand they became indistinguishable. And Harvey had no account of why the blood needed to flow rapidly through the body: he could merely show that it appeared to do so. For Aristotle and Galen scientific knowledge always included the understanding of what they called 'final' causes; that is to say, the purpose served by any natural process. Yet Harvey asked his readers to accept that the blood circulated as he described without being able to explain why it did so.

Harvey's argument depended on four key perceptions. In the order, perhaps, in which they occurred to him, they are: the valves in the veins, the movement of the heart, the quantity of blood leaving the heart, and the evidence that blood in the body was in continuous and unidirectional movement. The valves in the veins had been discovered by Hieronymus Fabricius, a Paduan anatomist whose lectures Harvey had attended while studying medicine at Padua. The only illustration in *De Motu Cordis* is a straightforward copy of one from Fabricius's *De Venarum Ostiolis* (1603). It shows how if you apply a light ligature to the arm you can make the veins stand out and can actually see the valves in them. Moreover you can press the blood along the vein in one direction but not in the other—the valve effectively blocks all flow away from the heart. Fabricius had failed to understand the significance of this simple experiment. He believed that the valves in the veins prevented blood from pooling in the extremities of the body; but Harvey recognized that what they really showed was that the blood could flow through the veins in only one direction. Realdo Colombo (d. 1559) had already argued that there was a unidirectional flow from right ventricle to left atrium, the pulmonary transit, and Harvey was acquainted with Colombo's work, although if he was indebted to it he never acknowledges the fact.

Second, close study of the exposed beating heart in animals convinced Harvey that Galen had misinterpreted the heart's action: when Galen thought it was contracting it was actually expanding, and vice versa. Harvey watched the heart more closely than Galen had been able to by studying its movement in slow motion in dying mammals and in cold-blooded creatures. An important consequence of this discovery was that Harvey could now see that the heart beats in synchrony with the pulse in the arteries, rather than, as Galen had believed, the two beats being out of step. This opened the way to recognizing that the pulse was merely the heartbeat reflected in the arteries.

Third, Harvey saw that if blood was forced out of the heart on each beat, then large quantities of blood must flow through the arteries; and if the valves in the heart, like those in the veins, were efficient, then the flow here too must be unidirectional. The consequence was that blood must flow through the system much more rapidly than it could be produced. Where was it coming from and where was it going? The only possible answer was that there was some mechanism for recycling it, that it was going round in a circle. Galen had already argued that arteries and veins were connected at their extremities, for

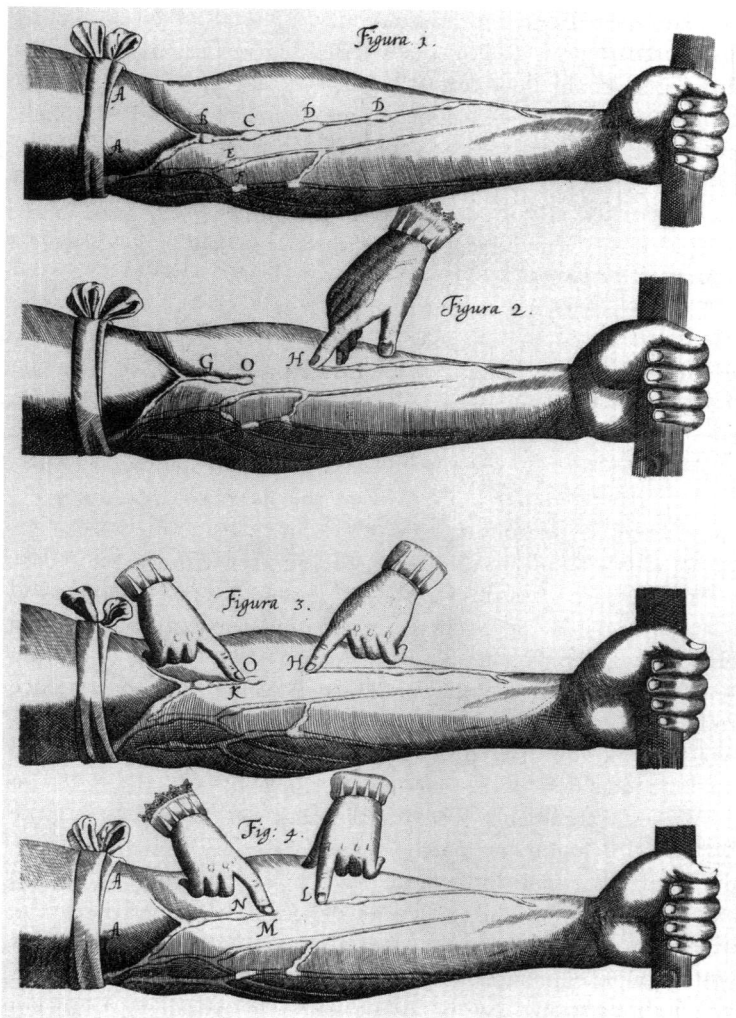

18. The illustration of the valves in the veins from Harvey's *De Motu Cordis*.

he knew that if one cut an artery all the blood would be drained out of the veins as well as the arteries. Harvey had only to argue that blood could flow through from arteries to veins by hidden connections to have an account of the circulation of the blood. He had a model in Aristotle's account of the circulation of water: water evaporates, falls as rain, seeps through the ground, runs in rivers to the sea, evaporates, and so on. Parts of this process—evaporation and percolation—are invisible, but one can tell they are taking place, for otherwise the rivers would eventually run dry.

Fourth, Harvey appealed to a number of key experiments where one could see this process at work. One had only to cut an artery to see the blood shoot out, and to see that the power of the jet reflected the rhythm of the heartbeat. Where Galenists had taken this copious flow to be a sign of the body's response to injury, Harvey took the cut in the artery wall as exposing what was going on anyway: the blood flowing rapidly under pressure from the heartbeat. Moreover, the blood always came from the side of the cut closest to the heart if one cut an artery, and from the side furthest from the heart if one cut a vein: Galen knew that this was the case, but he had no explanation for it, and in fact it is impossible to explain until one recognizes that the blood flows in only one direction. Again, when Harvey ligated the vein in the back of a snake, he could see the vein between the ligature and the heart being progressively emptied of blood as the blood was pumped through the heart into the arteries: here was the unidirectional flow of the blood made visible.

Harvey's arguments were simple and, he thought conclusive. But the first argument merely restated Fabricius's discoveries, and the third was essentially hypothetical. It was his second and fourth arguments that introduced new evidence, and both of these were dependent on experiments on living animals. Harvey's book begins with a couple of prefaces, an introduction, and a first chapter, subtitled 'the author's strong reasons for writing'. He gets down to serious business in chapter 2: 'The nature of the heart's movement, gauged from dissection of living animals'. Chapter 3 is entitled: 'The nature of the movement of the arteries, gauged from dissection of living animals'. Chapter 4: 'The nature of the movement of the heart and of the auricles [i.e. atria], gauged from dissection of living animals'. Without the dissection of living animals (the word *vivisection* was not invented until 1702, so that when Harvey discusses 'dissection' one always has to check whether he is dissecting the living or the dead—translations, such as the one I use, which employ the word 'vivisection' are anachronistic) Harvey would have had no argument.

Vivisection was not new with Harvey. Galen had practised vivisection: one of his favourite public demonstrations was to show that the voice was controlled by the brain not (as Aristotelians believed) by the heart; by slipping loops of thread around the inter-costal nerves he could deprive a squealing pig of its capacity to make a sound, and then restore its voice to it. Vesalius's successors in Padua had engaged in an extended programme of dissection and vivisection in animals. It is sometimes said that Vesalius himself merely echoes Galen when writing about vivisection and did not perform vivisec-tions himself; but the final chapter of the *De Fabrica* (which only appeared in English translation in 2003) makes it clear that Vesalius thought it best to accompany the dissection of a human corpse with the vivisection of an animal to show the parts of the body in oper-ation. Ideally one should use a pregnant bitch so that one could show the unborn puppies struggling to breathe as soon as the placental blood supply was cut off. Vesalius is perfectly clear that vivisection is a form of torture (the bitch is *cruciata*, crucified or tortured), but he delights in what it makes visible. Since his book is about the *human* body there is little place in it for an extended discussion of vivisection; but the opening illustration of the *Fabrica* shows the tools employed in dissection laid out on a vivisectionist's table (complete with ropes for tying down a struggling animal), while large initial Q shows a boar being vivisected and small initial Q shows a dog being vivisected. In employing vivisection Harvey was following in a distinguished tradition—the most striking advances in the understanding of human anatomy had taken place when Herophilus and Erasistratus had vivisected human beings.

It is easy to assume that Harvey was doing something funda-mentally new, and that it was that which made his discovery possible. Translations of Harvey frequently use the word 'experiment' and so it

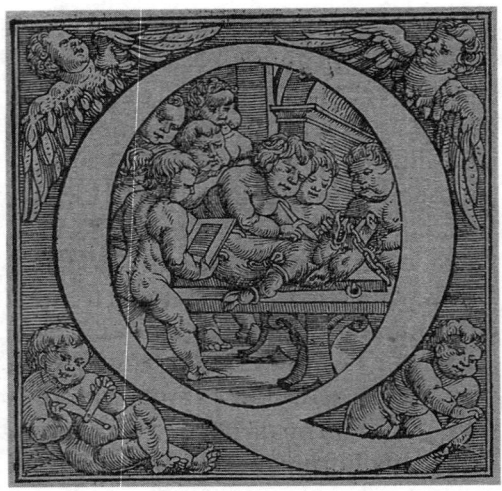

19. Large initial letter Q, showing the vivisection of a boar, from the 1555 edition of Vesalius's *De Fabrica*.

would seem obvious that Harvey was using a modern, experimental method. But in Latin the word *experimentum* normally means 'experience' rather than 'experiment' and it is not clear that there is anything new about Harvey's appeal to experience—Galen too had performed 'experiments'. Often one finds Harvey simply following in Galen's footsteps, as here in the Introduction:

> If one performed Galen's experiment, and incised the trachea of a still living dog, forcibly filling its lungs with air by means of bellows, and ligated them strongly in the distended position, one would find, on rapidly opening up the chest, a great deal of air in the lungs right out to their outermost coat, but no trace of such in the vein-like artery or in the left ventricle of the heart.

Had Harvey been an admirer of the new science, one would have expected him also to approve of Francis Bacon, whom later generations were to regard as the founder of the new empiricist scientific method. This was far from the case. John Aubrey reports that Harvey had been 'physician to the Lord Chancellor Bacon, whom he esteemed much for his wit and style; but would not allow him to be a great philosopher. Said he to me: "He writes philosophy like a Lord Chancellor" (speaking in derision).'

Failing a new experimental method, we might assume that what is new is Harvey's comparative approach, for he studies the heart not only in men and dogs, but also in snakes, frogs, and fishes, and even in the mammalian foetus within the womb (where the blood is spared a pointless journey to the as yet non-functional lungs by taking a short cut from the right to the left side of the heart via an opening, the foramen ovale, which closes shortly after birth). But Galen had conducted numerous vivisectional experiments, frequently exposing the heart in living animals; and he had studied the heart not only in men, apes, and dogs, but also in elephants and larks, in snakes and fishes. He had even experimented on the blood flow of unborn mammalian foetuses and knew about the *foramen ovale*. In any case, the idea of comparative anatomy goes back to Aristotle.

It is tempting to argue that it was much easier for Harvey to think in mechanical terms than it was for Galen. Notoriously Harvey discovered that the heart is a pump; it is characteristic of seventeenth-century scientists, not ancient Greeks and Romans, we might think, to see nature in terms of machines. It is true that in *De Motu Cordis* Harvey compares the heart to clockwork or to the firing mechanism of a flintlock pistol, mechanisms of which Galen had no knowledge. But in *De Motu Cordis* Harvey never compares the heart to a pump: it was only many years later that the sight of a pump on a simple fire engine led him first, in 1649, to compare the heart to a pump, and the arteries to hoses. Aristotle had compared the heart to a bellows, which establishes a unidirectional flow through efficient valves, so Galen could easily have constructed in his mind's eye an adequate mechanical model of the heart. There was no fundamental obstacle preventing him from seeing that the heart functioned as a pump.

Again, it has been argued that quantification is characteristic of seventeenth-century scientists who brought about a new marriage between mathematics and physics, and that it is this which makes it possible for Harvey to puzzle over the amount of blood pumped through the heart and where it goes. In fact the key texts of the new quantitative natural science had yet to be published in 1628 (Galileo's *Dialogue on the Two Chief Systems of the World* appeared in 1632); moreover Galen had puzzled, in exactly the same way as Harvey puzzled over the flow of blood, over the amount of liquid which flowed through the kidneys. There was no fundamental obstacle preventing Galen from quantifying the flow of blood through the arteries.

In fact, no matter how hard you try (and I say this with feeling, as this is a personal admission of defeat) there is no way of identifying a difference of method or of intellectual equipment that distinguishes Harvey from Galen. Modern scholarship on Harvey is divided between those who think Harvey was a modern and those who think he was an 'ancient'; the simple answer is that if Harvey is a modern then so too is Galen. Why then did Galen fail to discover the circulation of the blood? A wonderfully learned and scholarly book, C. R. S. Harris's *The Heart and the Vascular System in Ancient Greek Medicine*, has been written to answer this question. In 455 closely printed pages Harris conclusively demonstrates (against the claims of some scholars) that Galen had no knowledge of the circulation of the blood; but he is still unable to provide any satisfactory account of why such knowledge was unavailable to Galen.

In short, there was no major cultural or intellectual gap between Harvey's world and Galen's. Where Vesalius's achievements depended entirely on the new technology of the printing press, Harvey's discovery could easily have taken place in a manuscript culture. The experimental method, comparative anatomy, mechanical models, quantification, and vivisection are familiar to Galen just as they are to Harvey. What makes this story even more complicated is that Galen was not always mistaken when Harvey claimed that he was. From Vesalius on, anatomists had puzzled over Galen's claim that there were fine tubes between the left and right ventricles through which blood could seep. Harvey's argument in part depended on denying the existence of such tubes, and yet they do exist—a fact that most modern histories of science refuse to acknowledge. Again, in a famous experiment copied from Erasistratus, Galen had attached a tube to a hole cut into the wall of an artery; below the tube, he said,

rebutting Erasistratus, the pulse ceased to exist, which Galen interpreted as evidence that the pulse was a contraction in the wall of the
artery. Harvey failed to discuss this experiment in *De Motu Cordis*, but
in a reply to his critics he said that Galen's experiment was almost
impossible to perform because of haemorrhaging. Nevertheless if one
did perform it one found that the pulse occurred below as well as
above the insertion point of the tube, evidence that it was caused by
the flow of blood, not by the artery wall. Attempts to repeat this
experiment, from the seventeenth century to the present day, have
produced equivocal and contrasting results: there is experimental
support for Galen as well as for Erasistratus and Harvey.

It is very hard to fault Galen's powers of observation, even if we
now prefer Harvey's explanations to Galen's. Galen, for example,
describes tying off the two carotid arteries in an animal in order to
prove that vital spirits reached the brain through the nose, and not just
through the blood. The animal survived and continued to function.
Surely Galen had botched his experiment? In the late seventeenth
century Thomas Willis discovered what is now called 'the circle of
Willis', a network of blood-vessels which ensures that even if a carotid
artery is blocked, blood still reaches the whole of the brain; both
carotid arteries can even be blocked, and a supply of blood can reach
the brain through the vertebral artery. Whether that supply could be
adequate, and whether Galen had botched his experiment, is a moot
point: one medical textbook expresses the view that obstruction of
both carotids in a human would 'probably not be compatible with
survival'; the pathophysiology of death by strangulation continues to
be controversial, but obstruction to the veins may well be as important as obstruction to the carotid arteries.

Perhaps if there had been a continuing tradition of vivisection after
Galen, an ancient Roman would have discovered the circulation of
the blood some fourteen hundred years before Harvey; certainly once
Vesalius had rediscovered Galen's techniques it took only a century to
establish first the pulmonary transit, then the valves in the veins, and
finally the circulation of the blood. The important thing to recognize
is that, even if an ancient Roman had discovered the circulation of the
blood, it would have made virtually no difference to the history of

medicine. For Harvey's revolutionary discovery had only limited implications for medical therapy. The discovery that there was one unified circulatory system meant that there was little point in worrying, as doctors were busily doing in the time of Vesalius, about where one should draw blood, as blood drawn from any vein would affect the system as a whole (nevertheless, doctors continued to debate this question in the nineteenth century). And Harvey's account of circulation made it easier to understand how drugs and poisons could work on the body as a whole, easier too to understand how to use a tourniquet in phlebotomy. But Harvey had no intention of questioning traditional medical therapies: he relied on the worthless therapies of bloodletting, purges, and emetics just as much as all the other disciples of Galen. He claimed to have a better understanding of how traditional therapies worked, not to be offering new ones. Harvey had no intention of transforming the practice of medicine; he intended merely to correct a limited topic in medical theory.

Harvey's new physiology, I have argued, owed everything to vivisection: it is this, not the experimental method, the mechanical model, or quantification, which made his advances possible. Not surprisingly, what people made of Harvey's work depended on what they thought of vivisection. Harvey's critics—Primrose (1630), Worm (1632), Parigiano (1635), Leichner (1646), Riolan (1648)—all argued that vivisection could tell one nothing about what happened in a healthy animal, and that it was unacceptably cruel. His supporters— Walaeus (1640), Conring (1646), Glisson (1653)—all copied his vivisectional experiments and were convinced by them. Riolan is an instructive case in point: he turned reluctantly and halfheartedly to vivisection, and ended up supporting a modified and deeply compromised theory of the circulation of the blood.

Harvey's most important reply to his critics was his *Excercitatio Anatomica de Circulatione Sanguinis* of 1649, which consists of two essays in reply to Riolan. The second is a sustained reply to 'those who cry out that I have striven after the empty glory of vivisections'. His response is to urge his readers to engage in vivisections themselves. 'All these things you can see in some fairly long artery, such as

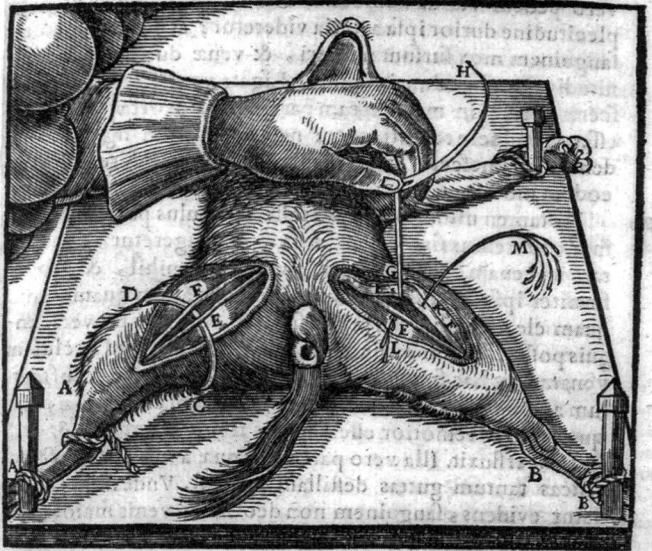

FIGURÆ EXPLICATIO.

A. *Crus canis dextrum.*   B. *Crus canis sinistrum.*

C. D. *Ligatura subiecta arteriæ & venæ, qua femur firmiter constringitur, expressa in dextro crure, ne literarum linearumque confusio in sinistro crure spectatorem posset turbare.*

E. *Arteria cruralis.*   F. *Vena cruralis.*

G. *Filum quo constricta est vena & est elevata.*

H. *Acus, cui filum est traiectum.*

I. *Venæ pars superior & detumescens.*

K. *Venæ pars inferior à ligatura intumescens.*

L. *Guttæ sanguinis, quæ, é superiori parte venæ vulnerata, sensim distillant.*

M. *Rivulus sanguinis, qui, inferiori venæ parte vulnerata, continuo exilit.*

F 2   vero

20. Vivisection of a dog from J. Walaeus, *Epistola Prima de Motu Chyli et Sanguinis* (1647).

the carotid, that you have cut. You will be able to take it between your fingers and to regulate the outflow of blood, exploring as you wish the increase and decrease, and loss and recovery, of pulsation . . .' As for Riolan, he only has to engage in 'a simple experiment' to discover that he is wrong to deny circulation in the mesenteric veins:

> In a vivisection, ligate the portal vein near the visceral part of the liver. You will see, from the swelling up of the veins below the ligature, that the same thing is happening as occurs in the administration of a phlebotomy from the placing of a ligature on the arm, revealing the passage of the blood at that point.

In the 1970s the Royal Society made a film for schools that reproduced Harvey's vivisections. I have met two people who were shown it at school; both told me that they could not bear to watch it all, and that some of their co-students fainted.

Harvey was prepared to accept that the final proof of his arguments rested on vivisection. In a letter to one of his critics, Casper Hofman, he writes: 'since you crave ocular evidence [of] the circulation of the blood . . . I now declare to you that I have also seen it clearly with my own eyes, and that I have very often demonstrated it by repeated vivisections to very clear-sighted folk'. All Hofman need do is allow Harvey to perform a demonstration for him, or else 'investigate by your own efforts in dissection' (by which, of course, is meant *vivisection*). This is what Harvey's sympathetic readers did. Thus the philosopher John Locke devised in the 1650s his own simple experiment to prove *circulatio sanguinis*: 'take a frog [and] strip [i.e. skin] it: you may see the circulation of blood if you hold him up against the sun'.

In the course of medical discussions such as those provoked by Harvey's *De Motu Cordis* something very strange happened to the English language. The word *autopsy* (from a Latin neologism, *autopsia*) originally meant to see with your own eyes; but slowly people lost track of its original meaning and began to use it, quite inappropriately, to mean a post-mortem dissection. When Harvey says the evidence for the circulation of the blood consists of 'autopsy or probable proof' is he using 'autopsy' to refer to 'ocular evidence' or to dissection? Either way, the vivisectionist's table had become the paradigmatic experimental space where nature was exposed to view.

The year before the publication of Harvey's *De Motu Cordis*, an Italian anatomist had announced the discovery of the lacteals in a vivisected dog. Not surprisingly, as Harvey's arguments became generally accepted (from the 1650s), experiments on living animals became the norm in biological research. The result was the discovery of the thoracic duct and the lymphatics. Boyle's vacuum pump experiments of 1659 showed that animals such as birds, shrews, snakes, and kittens could no more survive in a vacuum than could naked flames. From 1656 to 1666, Christopher Wren (an anatomist as well as architect), Thomas Willis (who published *The Anatomy of the Brain* in 1664), and Richard Lower experimented with transfusing various liquids into animals, beginning with poisons and ending up with blood. Willis, for example, injected dyes into living animals in order to stain the blood vessels. Nor were their experiments confined to animals. In 1657 the French Ambassador offered Wren 'an inferior domestic of his that deserved to have been hanged'—though the experiment was abandoned when the servant fainted on the sight of the equipment to be used! In 1666 Lower transfused blood from a lamb into a harmless madman, Arthur Coga. (The directors of the insane asylum of Bedlam had earlier refused to supply any of the inmates for experimental purposes.) Coga survived, but not surprisingly, he was not cured of insanity. Shortly afterwards a similar experiment in France resulted in a fatality, and blood transfusions involving humans were for a considerable time abandoned: in the mid-nineteenth century Lister would sometimes offer a transfusion to patients facing death, though how many lives were saved by this means I do not know.

The first high point for vivisection was the period 1664–8, when some ninety experiments were reported to the Royal Society, and some thirty conducted in front of its assembled members. In 1664 Robert Hooke, the Royal Society's professional experimentalist, performed a revised version of the Galen/Harvey experiment involving pumping up the lungs of a vivisected dog. Where Galen and Harvey had blocked the windpipe when the lungs were inflated, Hooke attached a pair of bellows to the opened windpipe, and showed that he could keep the dog alive as long as he pumped air into the lungs, even if he removed the rib cage—thus showing that those (including Harvey) who thought that the mechanical movement of the rib cage played some vital role in sustaining life were quite wrong. For the most part, Hooke's experiment was met with praise; but Hooke himself was horrified by what he had done. He announced that 'I shall hardly be induced to make any further trials of this kind because of the torture of the creature; but certainly the enquiry would be very noble, if we could find any way so to stupefy the creature, as that it might not be sensible, which I fear there is hardly any opiate will perform.' Around the same time, in *Micrographia* (1665), he praised the use of the microscope as enabling one to look at nature 'acting according to her usual course and way, undisturbed, whereas when we endeavour to pry into her secrets by breaking open the doors upon her, and dissecting and mangling creatures whilst there is life yet within them, we find her indeed at work, but put into such disorder by the violence offered' that we cannot tell if the results are of any significance. This debate persists.

Despite his reservations, in 1667 Hooke agreed to perform (he was after all an employee), with Lower's assistance, a more advanced form of the thoracic experiment in front of the Royal Society. This time an incision was to be made in the dog's lungs so that the air pumped in by the bellows would flow straight through them, and two bellows were to be put to work so that the flow of air was continuous—the lungs would thus remain entirely stationary. The experiment was carried out, and proved that movement in the lungs was not necessary to their function. John Evelyn, the diarist, was present and found the experiment 'of more cruelty than pleased me'. In a later version of the experiment, Lower opened the pulmonary vein, and showed that blood returning from the lungs to the heart was already an arterial red.

It is sometimes said that people in the seventeenth century had no notion of cruelty to animals, and Descartes even argued that animals are mere machines, incapable of feeling pain. It is also said that there was so much cruel treatment of one human being by another in the seventeenth century that what was done by the vivisectionists to animals would scarcely have seemed horrendous. But Hooke and Evelyn were not alone in finding certain vivisections repugnant. The Danish naturalist Nicholas Steno wrote to Thomas Bartholin in 1661 expressing his dismay at the vivisecting of dogs: 'I must admit that it is not without abhorrence that I torture them with such prolonged pain.' And after the 1690s, anti-vivisectionist sentiments were commonly expressed in France and England. Modern historians of science celebrate the 'discoveries' of Wren, Willis, Lower, Boyle, and Hooke: the first intravenous injections, the first blood transfusions, the first anatomy of the brain, the first account of the physiology of respiration. It is worth stressing that, as with Harvey's discovery of the circulation of the blood, this extended programme of animal vivisection had no therapeutic benefits. Not a single life was saved, not a single illness abbreviated.

Historians have been very reluctant to face the fact that vivisection (and not something apparently harmless, such as 'the experimental method') was the true foundation of the new physiology. Similarly, they have sought to play down the extent to which the new anatomy, which arose out of dissection, depended on activities (such as the boiling up of bodies) that even the leading participants felt were abhorrent. Above all, they have sought to downplay the fact that all this new knowledge was entirely useless, in that it led to only minor and marginal changes in therapy. For example Willis, the first specialist in brain anatomy, treated epilepsy with emetics to induce vomiting, with leeches, with peony roots and wolves' livers, and with amulets filled with mistletoe. He had (to borrow his own words) 'slain so many vicitims, whole hecatombs almost of all animals, in the anatomical court', and yet had nothing practical to show for it. Still, his experiments stood him in good stead: 'He became so noted, and so infinitely resorted to, for his practice,' wrote Anthony Wood, 'that never any physician before went beyond him, or got more money yearly than he.'

7

THE INVISIBLE WORLD

Historians generally shy away from might-have-beens, but the argument of this chapter is that something very strange happened in late seventeenth-century science: an intellectual revolution that should have taken place failed to occur. In the 1670s and 1680s the microscope made possible a series of major discoveries. These discoveries should have been followed by others; yet they were not. Instead the microscope was abandoned as a significant tool for biological research; not until the 1830s did serious research recommence. It used to be thought that there was a straightforward explanation for this: the microscopes of the 1830s were much better than those of the 1680s. Now we know that this was not the case. So what went wrong?

The telescope and microscope were invented simultaneously, and probably by the same person, in Holland between 1608 and 1610. News of the new devices reached Galileo, whose *Sidereal Messenger* (1610), based on his discoveries with the telescope, immediately began the revolution in astronomy. Galileo himself constructed microscopes (the word is first used of one of his instruments, in 1625); but the first detailed account of the interior construction of a living being based on the use of a microscope did not appear until 1644, in Giambattista Odierna's *L'occhio della mosca*, or *The Fly's Eye*. Here is the first mystery: where the relevance of the telescope to astronomy was recognized immediately, the relevance of the microscope to biology and medicine was not recognized for a generation or two.

It is not until the 1660s and 1670s that the microscope began seriously to be put to use, in Italy, England, and Holland, with a host of studies by the five great microscopists of the seventeenth century. The first was Marcello Malpighi, who pioneered the use of the microscope to explore minute biological structures, beginning with

De Pulmonibus, On the Lungs (1661) and more or less ending with *De Ovo Incubato, The Incubation of the Egg* (1675), based on the microscopic study of the incubation of chickens' eggs. Classical medicine had assumed that liver, spleen, kidneys, lungs were essentially made out of congealed blood and were therefore formless lumps of material; Malpighi showed that these organs had complicated internal structures. Next came Robert Hooke's *Micrographia* (1665), which had an enormous impact with the public because of its wonderful illustrations, including a double-page pull-out image of a louse. Then came Jan Swammerdam's *Historiae Generalis Insectorum* (1669). Swammerdam was a brilliant researcher who died young. He was painfully torn between the belief that the study of the creation was a way of glorifying the creator and a fear that to concentrate one's attention on the material world was to lose touch with spiritual realities. In 1673 came the first publications of Nehemiah Grew (an Englishman who did careful studies of the internal structures of plants) and above all of the great Antoni van Leeuwenhoek, who in the space of a few years discovered the red blood cells, and a new world of microscopic living creatures, including the spermatozoa.

Between 1661 and 1691 more was discovered in biology than in any other generation since the death of Aristotle, yet in 1692 Hooke complained that the serious use of the microscope had been almost completely abandoned. This, the decline of microscopy, is the second mystery. Of the famous microscopists only Leeuwenhoek was still at work: he died in 1723. Swammerdam had died in 1680; Grew published nothing on biology after 1684; and Malpighi had published his final work in 1689. These pioneers had no successors; there was, Hooke lamented, no money to be made by microscopy. The same complaint was made by Leeuwenhoek towards the end of his life, in 1715. He reported that in the university town of Leiden many students had taken up microscopy and had learnt how to make microscopes, but in the end all had abandoned this line of work. There was no money in it.

The third mystery lies in the fact that the microscope did not establish itself as a serious tool for scientific research until the 1830s, when the problem of chromatic aberration (long believed insoluble) was finally overcome and the microscope began for the first time to be commonly used in medical education. Chromatic aberration makes rainbows possible: different colours are refracted at different angles, so that each time you pass light through a lens you create a halo of colours around the object you are looking at, eventually obscuring it from sight. Chromatic aberration had imposed severe limits on the magnifying power and resolution of microscopes constructed, on the model of the telescope, out of several lenses, so that there was little progress in the design of compound microscopes between 1610 and 1830. Consequently nothing could seem more straightforward: the answer to our puzzle is that early microscopy failed because of the inherent limits of the instruments at the disposal of the first researchers—except for the fact that there were two entirely different types of microscope in use in the period before 1830.

Malpighi, Hooke and Grew relied primarily on compound microscopes; Swammerdam and Leeuwenhoek relied primarily on simple microscopes. Where compound microscopes use two or more lenses, simple microscopes use only one and are much less affected by chromatic aberration. In order to get high magnifications this single lens has to be very sharply curved: a simple microscope uses a tiny bead of glass, and as a result the focal length is incredibly short. The object looked at, the lens, and the human eye have all to be within a very short distance of each other. In the case of Leeuwenhoek's best surviving lens the object has to be placed 0.5 mm from the lens, and the lens has to be virtually up against the eyeball. Because the object has to be held up to the eye it can really only be illuminated from behind, which makes it difficult to look properly at objects which are not semi-transparent. Through a tiny lens one can see only a minute area at a time. The simple microscope thus has very marked technical limitations. In addition, learning to use it is far from straightforward. In 1986 an article in the *Proceedings of the Royal Microscopical Society* reproduced photographs taken through the lens of Leeuwenhoek's best surviving simple microscope: the point was to show that the images were hopelessly blurred and that the simple microscope could never have been a serious tool for biological research.

Then in 1991 Brian J. Ford published a remarkable book, *The Leeuwenhoek Legacy*. One of the arguments of the historians of microscopy had been that the specimens prepared by seventeenth-century microscopists must have been hopelessly crude. Ford found in the papers of the Royal Society a collection of specimens sent by Leeuwenhoek to London. It was easy to photograph them with modern microscopes, and to put the resulting photographs side by side with modern photographs of the same type of material, and thus to show conclusively that Leeuwenhoek, working with a cut-throat razor, was able to produce specimens every bit as good as those produced in a modern laboratory. But Ford achieved something even more remarkable. By fitting one of Leeuwenhoek's lenses into a modern camera he was able to overcome the focusing problems that had bedevilled his predecessors.

The best of Leeuwenhoek's surviving lenses has a magnification of x266, and resolves down to 1.35 microns (or micrometers or μ m): 0.2 micron is the theoretical limit for an optical, as opposed to electron, microscope; a human hair is about 100 microns, and bacteria are 2–5 microns. Using this lens, Ford was able to produce photographs that are closely comparable in quality to those taken through the lenses of a modern compound microscope. After his work there can be no doubt that Leeuwenhoek's microscopes were comparable in power to those of the 1830s and 1840s, which were capable of resolving down to about 1 micron. By comparison, the earliest good-quality compound microscopes to survive, from around 1700, magnify x150 and resolve down to 2.5 microns, and medical students now work with microscopes that resolve down to half a micron. As late as 1827 von Baer produced the first description of the mammalian ovum using a simple microscope, and in 1833, when cell theory had yet to be constructed, Robert Brown identified what we now know as the nucleus of plant cells using a simple microscope. From 1669 to 1827 the best microscopes were simple microscopes.

In 1960, when I was 8, I was something of an expert myself in the use of simple microscopes. Because my parents lived abroad I was home-schooled, and my mother was supplied with suitable materials by the PNEU. (I remember the initials clearly, but what did they stand

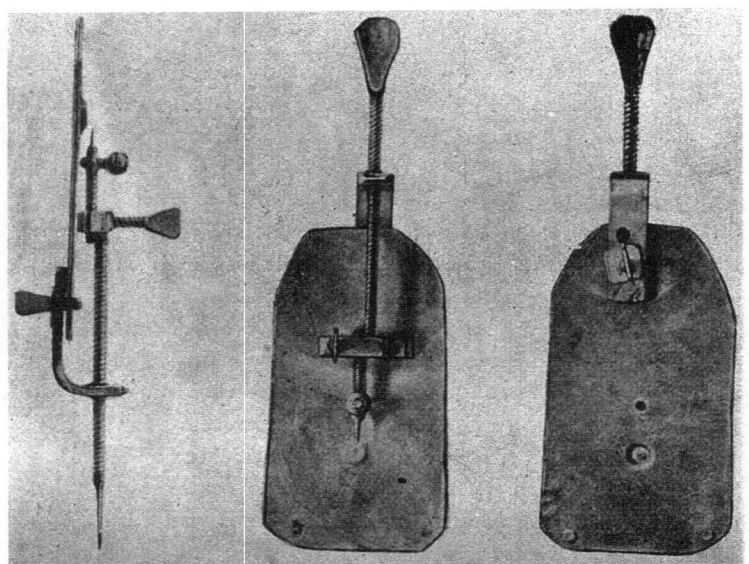

21. One of Leeuwenhoek's microscopes. The specimen would be placed on the needle in front of the tiny lens (near the top in the lefthand image, and the bottom in the central and righthand images).

for? The Parents National Education Union?) Years later I discovered that my knowledge of the history of art was based almost entirely on illustrations of pictures from the Kenwood Gallery in London which had evidently been the PNEU's chief source. My knowledge of biology was based almost entirely on a perfectly functional simple microscope supplied by the PNEU with a collection of samples. I mention this because Brian Ford has explored the modern history of the simple microscope, but does not seem to have come across these mass-produced educational implements with which I and my contemporaries were able to replicate some of Leeuwenhoek's discoveries. But the very qualities which made the simple microscope suitable for an 8 year old—its cheapness, its ease of manufacture, its inherently low-tech design—made it seem a toy rather than a scientific instrument. The failure of microscopy to establish itself before the 1830s has a good deal to do with the low status of the simple microscope. Leeuwenhoek seems to have been aware of this problem: so simple and cheap were his microscopes to produce that he made some five hundred of them, all for his own personal use. But many of them he plated in silver or gold in order to give them a prestige they would otherwise have lacked.

Leeuwenhoek was acutely aware of questions of status because his own was so low. He was by trade a draper, and then an employee of the city of Delft. He had no academic education, and spoke, wrote, and read only Dutch. As a result he knew of the work of other scientists only through conversations and through having their books explained to him by those capable of reading them. Initially he was reluctant to publish his discoveries, and at first he repeatedly asked his readers to take into consideration who he was, in other words his humble origins. Throughout his life as a researcher he mixed uncomfortably with those better educated, wealthier, and with more polished manners than his own. He never wrote a book; all he produced were letters. Yet, between 1673 and 1723 more than a hundred of these letters (or extracts from them) were published in the *Transactions* of the Royal Society, and during his lifetime collections of his letters were also made and published in Dutch and Latin. If Leeuwenhoek had only a limited knowledge of the work of other scientists, they had every opportunity to know about his work.

The failure of the nascent scientific community to recognize the significance of Leeuwenhoek's discoveries is the most important of all the mysteries involved in the history of microscopy. It was not until the 1660s that the power of the simple microscope was first recognized; had the importance of Leeuwenhoek's work been understood there would have been no failure of the simple microscope to establish itself as a serious research tool, and there would have been no decline in microscopic research after the 1680s. Leeuwenhoek's discoveries represented the first real opportunity to transform medical practice since bloodletting, purging, and emetics had established themselves as the key therapies within the Greek tradition of medicine more than two thousand years before. Had the significance of what Leeuwenhoek had discovered been understood, there would have been no need to wait until the middle of the nineteenth century for the revolution in medicine from which we still benefit.

There is an important sense in which medical time stood still or even went backwards between Hooke's 1692 complaint that microscopy had been virtually abandoned and 1837, when Schwann formulated the germ theory of putrefaction. Conventional histories of medical knowledge, taking progress as their underlying (but generally unavowed) narrative, assume that if people change their minds they must do so for good reasons. They are incapable of giving a coherent account of eighteenth-century biology and medicine because the story cannot be told as a story of progress; it is rather a story of squandered opportunities, of wasted effort, of intellectual dead ends. It is a history of failure.

Three examples make this clear: the theory of reproduction; the theory of spontaneous generation; the theory of animate contagion. In 1672 Regnier de Graaf published *De Mulierum Organis, On Women's Organs*, in which, drawing on microscopic evidence, he refuted a fundamental principle of Aristotelian biology. For over two thousand years the assumption had been that the anatomy of men and women was fundamentally the same. Men were just produced under more favourable conditions than women—in Aristotelian terms, in hotter wombs. As a result their sexual organs were more developed and protruded from the body. Women had the same sexual organs, but they were folded inside the body. The penis thus corresponded to the vagina. It is easy to imagine that because the word *vagina* is Latin (meaning sheath, as in the sheath for a sword) the ancient Romans used the word to refer to a part of the female anatomy. But Greek, Roman, medieval, and Renaissance doctors used the same word for penis and vagina, and the same word for testicles and ovaries. Women had a penis and they had testicles.

Aristotle had sharply distinguished the roles of the sexes: in sexual congress, the man supplied the form, the woman the matter. Men were agents and women were passive. But Galen had taken the supposed similarity in the biological structure of men and women entirely seriously. Both men and women, he believed, had orgasms, and both produced semen—a theory that implied that women could not become pregnant without orgasm. It was the mixing of these semens that made conception possible. The difference between men and women was thus a matter of degree, not kind. This general theory survived the discovery of the clitoris by the other Columbus, Realdo Colombo (1516–59), though it was evident, particularly in hermaphrodites, that the clitoris bore a relationship of analogy to the penis. But the theory was destroyed by de Graaf, who showed that the internal structure of the male testicles (on which he had published a treatise in 1668, although Johannes van Horne claimed to have made the key discovery slightly earlier) was quite different from that of the female testicles. In fact, de Graaf argued, the female testicles were ovaries and must produce eggs. De Graaf immediately found himself involved in another bitter dispute over priority, this time with Swammerdam.

At once, one would have thought, efforts would have concentrated on trying to actually *see* a mammalian egg. But after the death of de Graaf (1673) and Swammerdam (1680) research stood still. In 1737 and 1738 when Swammerdam's unpublished manuscripts were finally published, more than fifty years after his death, they still represented entirely new knowledge, but did not contain any observation of the ovum, which had to wait until von Baer's work in 1827. Where in the late 1660s there had been a whole group of Dutch scientists— de Graaf, Swammerdam, Horne (d. 1670), Nicolaus Steno (d. 1686, who had discovered the ovaries of fish in 1667)—competing to be the first to make discoveries in this field, it took one hundred and fifty years to bring their work to a successful conclusion. In the meantime, in the world of biological research, time stood still.

Despite their failure to actually look for eggs, scientists between the 1680s and the 1830s generally took the view that plants, fish, and mammals all developed from eggs and that the new life existed preformed within the egg: we now call this *ovism*. Where for two thousand years, Aristotelians had held that new life comes into existence at conception, the dominant view from the late seventeenth century was that all new life implied new creation, and any act of creation involved a miracle. Rather than accepting that God was constantly working miracles, scientists preferred to argue that all life had been created by God when he created the world. What appeared to be new life was rather the development of existing life. Swammerdam showed that butterflies, which appeared to be new creatures born out of the pupa, in fact existed already in the caterpillar em; by dissection he could identify the presence of their organs within the caterpillar's body. So too the parts of the full-grown plant could be found within the seed, as Malpighi showed in 1675. The logical conclusion of this line of argument was that Eve had within her body the eggs which would develop into her children, and within those eggs were already preformed the eggs which would develop into her daughters' children, and so on, as in Russian dolls, each with a smaller doll nested within it. Eve thus contained nested within her ovaries every future human being, already created, already formed, merely awaiting development. Preformation was held to entail pre-existence.

There were obvious problems with this line of argument. It made it very difficult to explain why offspring sometimes took after their fathers: as early as 1683 Leeuwenhoek had noted that if you crossed large white female domestic rabbits with small grey male wild rabbits you always got small, grey rabbits; in 1752 Maupertuis showed that in human beings polydactylism (having six fingers, not five) is always inherited in the male line. It was hard to see how ovism could explain such cases where characteristics were inherited from the male. It also made it hard to understand how you could have hybrids, how a donkey and a horse could mate, for example, and produce a mule. Moreover, if all the parts of a creature existed in the egg, and merely developed rather than being constructed from nothing, how was it possible for some creatures to regenerate parts that had been lost? In 1688 Claude Perrault wrote a dissertation on the regeneration of lizards' tails. In 1712 René Antoine Ferchault de Réaumur pub-lished an account of the regeneration of crayfish claws. Worst of all, in 1741 Abraham Trembley showed that you could cut a polyp into a dozen pieces and it would turn into a dozen polyps. Was this not the creation of new living beings?

Leeuwenhoek used his rabbits to argue that the future creature existed preformed not in the egg but in the sperm (which he claimed to have been the first to observe through a microscope); thus off-spring took after their fathers, not their mothers. But fundamentally spermaticism (as Leeuwenhoek's alternative to ovism is called) was open to exactly the same objections as ovism. Throughout the eight-eenth century most biologists remained attached to ovism despite all the obvious difficulties, and despite the fact that they had no clear account of what sperm were for. (If anything: in 1785 Lazzaro Spallanzani claimed to have definitively shown that one could fertilize frog spawn with frog semen from which every spermatozoon had been removed.) Ovism remained dominant until the birth of cell theory in the 1830s, despite the fact that it could not explain Leeuwenhoek's rabbits, Perrault's lizards, or Trembley's polyps. Here, too, time stood still, for the evidence adduced by Trembley or Maupertuis in the 1740s and 1750s was not fundamentally different from that being produced by Leeuwenhoek and Perrault in the 1680s.

We see the same pattern when we turn to the most important of all the discoveries made by the first generation of microscopists, and the debates that arose out of it. In a letter to the Royal Society of 9 October 1676 Leeuwenhoek reported finding tiny micro-organisms far smaller than anything previously known to exist. He had found them in rainwater, in lake water, in canal water. He had found them in infusions of pepper and ginger (hence at first they were called *infusoria*). He had discovered a new, previously invisible world. Where previously microscopists had been looking at things they already knew existed—the eyes of flies, for example—Leeuwenhoek was now looking at creatures whose very existence had been unsuspected. Soon he was finding micro-organisms almost everywhere he looked: in the crud between his toes, in the guck between his teeth, in his faeces when he had diarrhoea. They were everywhere.

At first, using his low-powered compound microscope, Hooke in London was unable to replicate Leeuwenhoek's discovery. It was only in the summer of 1677, when he had constructed a simple micro-scope at Leeuwenhoek's direction, that he was able to see these new creatures and to show them to the assembled members of the Royal Society. The next year, Christiaan Huygens demonstrated them to the Académie des Sciences in Paris. By September 1679 however

Nicolaas Hartsoeker could report that 'French curiosity concerning the microscopes has disappeared entirely.' In England no one other than Leeuwenhoek published on micro-organisms until 1693 (when the subject was taken up again, perhaps in response to Hooke's complaint of 1692 that microscopes were unduly neglected). Around the same time, Huygens returned to work on them, but he was at the end of his life. It was not until 1718 that there was any sustained attempt to describe this new microscopic world. In that year Louis Joblot, a mathematician, painter, and sculptor who used simple microscopes, published his *Descriptions et usages de plusieurs nouveaux microscopes . . . avec de nouveaux observations*. He had no successors. It had taken forty years to do work which could have been completed within two or three, and still no one grasped the significance of what had been found.

The discovery of micro-organisms transformed two existing debates, over spontaneous generation and over the nature of contagious diseases. All conventional seventeenth-century biologists (even the very best amongst them, such as Harvey) believed that large numbers of creatures—mice, flies, fleas, bees—could be spontaneously generated under the right circumstances. Consequently there was little point in drawing a sharp line between the inanimate and the animate: every pile of grain was capable of generating a mouse, every warm body was capable of generating a flea. Swammerdam and Leeuwenhoek, however, were the first great opponents of the idea of spontaneous generation. Indeed Leeuwenhoek's friend Nicolaas Hartsoeker later said that, if Leeuwenhoek's researches had a purpose, that purpose was the refutation of spontaneous generation.

The subject of spontaneous generation was already a live one when modern microscopy began. In 1662 the Royal Society was conducting experiments to see if it could generate insects in closed vessels: it failed, and concluded that spontaneous generation did not occur. This group of experimenters did not however understand that insects only appeared where eggs had been laid: it assumed that the air was full of invisible, drifting insect *semina* (seeds). In 1668, Francesco Redi tried a variation of the same experiment: he failed to generate flies, wasps, ants, or other insects from a range of substances within

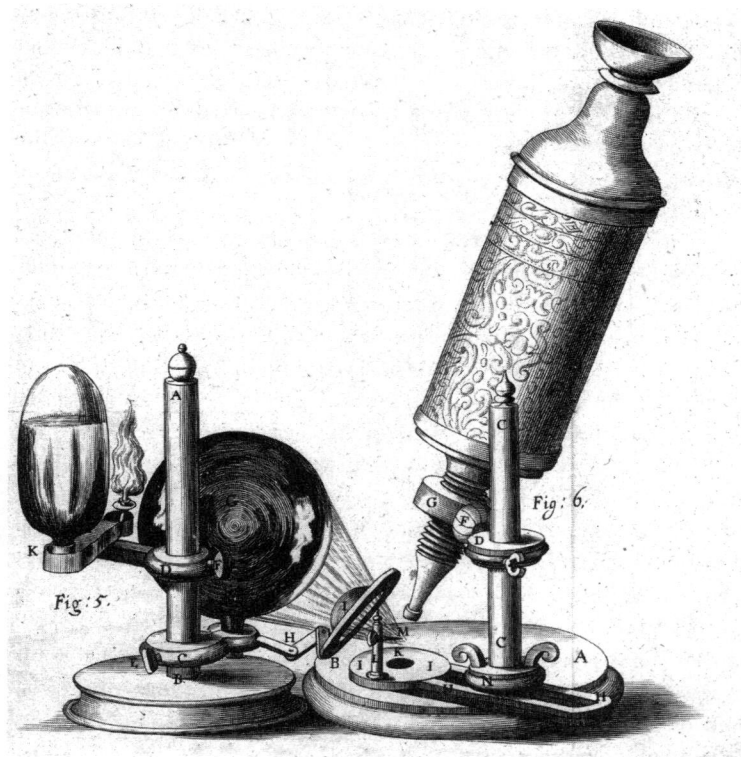

22. The compound miscroscope used by Hooke, as illustrated in his *Micrographia* (1665).

covered vessels, including buffalo, tiger, lamb, dog, and rabbit meat. He was, though, persuaded that worms in fruit and in the human intestine developed spontaneously—the origins of worms in fruit was to be resolved by Vallisnieri (1661–1730), but the life cycle of intestinal parasites was to remain a mystery until the work of Steenstrup (1842) and von Siebold (1852). In June 1680 Leeuwenhoek tried to extend Redi's experiments to see if micro-organisms would be generated in sealed environments containing rainwater, or ground pepper infused in water: he found that they were, but he suspected that this was because their eggs were already inside the sealed containers. In France, Louis Joblot demonstrated in 1707 that micro-organisms did not develop in a water and manure mixture that had been boiled for some time and then sealed. Further experiments convinced him that micro-organisms (like insects) developed from eggs floating in the air.

Crucial to the developing argument against spontaneous generation was the recognition that insects reproduced sexually. In 1668 Swammerdam discovered that what had always been taken to be the king bee was in fact a queen who laid eggs, and he went on to discover the sex organs of the male drones. In 1687 Leeuwenhoek demonstrated that the grain weevil came from a tiny worm rather than being spontaneously generated in its adult form. He went on to illustrate the male sex organs of the grain weevil, the grain moth, the flea, the louse, and even to discover the spermatozoa within the male louse (which were, strangely enough, no smaller than human spermatozoa). He also showed that common parasites, such as tapeworms, entered the body from outside and were not generated spontaneously from within. Meanwhile Malpighi was dissecting the sex organs of the female silkworm moth. From Aristotle on, biologists had believed that some creatures were capable both of spontaneous generation and of sexual reproduction, but Swammerdam, Leeuwenhoek, and Malpighi took the view that where they had demonstrated sexual reproduction they had disproved spontaneous generation. Consequently they felt sure that insects were never spontaneously generated, and Leeuwenhoek felt confident in extending this conclusion to micro-organisms.

Here too, though, time stood still. In 1707, Joblot thought he had decisive evidence in support of Leeuwenhoek. In 1748, John Turberville Needham, an Irish Catholic priest, claimed to have subjected a sealed flask containing gravy to prolonged high heat; yet after four days it was full of micro-organisms which had apparently been spontaneously generated. In 1765 another Catholic priest, Spallanzani, repeated Needham's experiment, this time sealing nineteen flasks by melting the glass and then boiling the gravy within them for an hour. If Needham's flasks had generated micro-organisms it was, he concluded, because the air within them had not been heated to a temperature high enough to kill off any eggs that might be floating in it. Spallanzani proceeded to do elaborate experiments to find out at what temperatures different types of organism, from bats to fleas, could survive. Needham and his supporters replied that Spallanzani, by heating the air, must have changed its nature, so that it was no longer capable of supporting life. Admit fresh air, and micro-organisms would immediately appear.

From 1707 until well into the nineteenth century versions of what was essentially the same experiment were repeated over and over again, with differing results. After Joblot, after Spallanzani, after Schwann (1837), even after Pasteur (1862) claimed to have refuted spontaneous generation the debate continued. In 1765 Heinrich August Wrisberg, in 1766 Otto von Münchausen, in 1767 Carl Linnaeus, in 1786 Otto Frederik Müller, in 1859 Felix Pouchet, in 1862 Jeffries Wyman (working at Harvard), in 1875 Henry Bastian: each claimed to have proof of spontaneous generation. For more than a century and a half the battle over the spontaneous generation of micro-organisms was fought, and essentially the same experiment was repeated with ever more complex variations. Here, too, time stood still.

The same is true of the debate over the nature of contagious diseases. Traditional medicine held that disease was caused by an imbalance in the humours. This was holistic medicine: to restore health one had to treat the individual, not the disease. There was nothing real about diseases as such, they were just symptoms of an underlying condition, and a wide variety of underlying conditions might produce the same symptoms, or the same underlying condition might manifest itself as several different symptoms. To treat his patient, the doctor had to understand his patient's individual patterns of response, and to recognize that a quite new set of symptoms might be a reflection of a continuing imbalance.

The Hippocratic authors had for the most part assumed that when whole communities were hit by plague this was because they all breathed the same air and drank the same water. Galenic medicine, however, placed much less emphasis on external environment as a cause of disease, leaving it much harder to understand why very different people—the young, the old, the fit, the frail—should suffer simultaneously from the same disease. By the Renaissance this issue was much more acute. The Black Death in 1348 was the first outbreak of bubonic plague in Western Europe, but outbreaks continued to recur into the late seventeenth century. Syphilis was, if not unknown, extremely rare in Europe before Columbus's voyages of exploration. These were diseases that appeared to have a life of their own, and to pass directly from one healthy individual to another.

In 1546 Girolamo Fracastoro published *De Contagione, et Contagiosis Morbis, et Eorum Curatione*, or *On Contagion*, in which he explored these peculiar 'contagious' diseases. Syphilis was clearly usually passed by close contact between two individuals, but plague seemed to have the capacity to lay dormant and then break out. Italian communes, ignoring Galenic and Hippocratic orthodoxy, had long practised quarantine to prevent the transmission of plague, and burnt the personal effects of those who died of plague. These measures seemed to work. But why? Fracastoro, probably drawing on passing remarks in Galen and a key passage in Lucretius, *De Rerum Natura* (*c.*56 BC), explored the ways in which a disease might enter a healthy body from the outside. It might be comparable to a poison, or it might be comparable to a seed, which could lie dormant, be carried by the wind, and then sprout when it found favourable conditions.

From Fracastoro on into the eighteenth century there is a continuous tradition of discussing the 'seeds' of disease. This early theory is often thought to be strikingly similar to the 'germ' theory later developed by Pasteur. But it is important to see the respects in which Fracastoro was not a germ theorist. Although he held that many diseases were normally transmitted from person to person by contagion, he also held that every disease, even syphilis, is capable of arising spontaneously within an individual or an environment if the conditions are right. He thus believed that diseases could be spontaneously generated. Second, he carefully avoided committing himself as to exactly what sort of thing it was that transmitted diseases, whether it was inanimate (like a poison) or animate (like a seed). His preferred term was *seminaria*, which is normally translated as 'germ', but a *seminaria* is a seed-bed; it is something out of which a seed sprouts. In order to be a proper 'germ' theory, a theory needs to both deny that diseases can generate spontaneously and insist that the agent of contagion is animate. Fracastoro fails these two tests, as for example does Gabriele Fallopio, in 1564, who argued that syphilis and phthisis were caused by the transmission of blood particles.

It would take a good deal of research to establish which of the supposed early germ theorists pass these tests. In 1650, August Hauptmann argued that diseases were caused by minute wormlets: this was the first appeal to the microscope in this context. In 1658 the Jesuit Athanasius Kircher argued that plague, leprosy, venereal disease, and elephantiasis were caused by a subvisible *effluvia animata*, and that putrefaction was caused by organisms visible only under a microscope. In 1664 Henry Power thought that plague was caused by living creatures in the air. In 1665 Ysbrand van Diemerbroeck thought that plague was caused by 'seeds'. In 1696 Johannes Paulitz, studying in Leiden, thought contagious seeds were everywhere. In 1700 Nicolas Andry de Boisregard believed invisible insects were the causes of disease.

In the history of disease theory 1711 marks an important moment, for scientists were able to observe the appearance in Europe, first of all in the Venetian territories, of a new disease of cattle, rinderpest. Carlo Francesco Cogrossi (one of Antonio Vallisnieri's pupils) argued in 1714 that it was an invisible micro-organism that was responsible for the new cattle plague: in reply Vallisnieri wondered whether there might be a way of poisoning such creatures. Cogrossi was clear about his intellectual debts: he appealed to Leeuwenhoek's discovery of micro-organisms, and to the work of Giovanni Bonomo, who had demonstrated in 1687 that the eggs of a tiny mite, visible only under the microscope, were responsible for scabies. Bonomo was an associate of Redi's, and Redi had formulated the concept of a parasite: Bonomo was showing that scabies was caused by minute parasites. Similar arguments to those of Cogrossi are to be found in Richard Bradley in 1718 and Benjamin Marten in 1720. In 1722 Thomas Fuller even tried to explain how one might acquire immunity to such creatures. The subject was sufficiently topical for an anonymous author, A.C.D., to claim in 1726 that he had discovered the little creatures that caused disease. Unfortunately his evidence was faked.

The examples given above represent a very incomplete list. Just how inattentive historians have been to this subject is well illustrated by a letter that almost every early modern medical historian has read, William Harvey's letter to Giovanni Nardi of 30 November 1653, in which Harvey discusses a book in which Nardi 'had attributed almost the same efficient cause to plague as I had ascribed to the generation of animals'. In the case of generation, Harvey says, it is difficult to understand how the semen conveys something of the male to the foetus, so that it takes after him.

> Yet I think it is equally difficult to understand how the essence of a pestilence or of leprosy can be communicated even to a distance by contact, especially through an intermediary such as the agency of woolen or linen clothes . . . How, I ask, can contagion, long dormant in things of that kind later emerge from them and that after a long interval, and produce something similar to itself even in another body?

Harvey scholars have noted that elsewhere Harvey compares contagion and generation, and Wilson is correct to say that Harvey 'was not supposing that seeds of plague that germinate in the human body were involved'.

But nobody has bothered to read Giovanni Nardi's 'learned comments on Lucretius', published in 1647, from which it immediately becomes apparent that Nardi was indeed thinking in terms of seeds of plague germinating in the human body. Why did Harvey not understand Nardi on this subject? Why was his response so beside the point? For certainly the point did elude him—in the theory of seeds of plague a seed was something that could be transported from one place to another, could be carried in clothes, could lie dormant, and then prove fertile. The answer would seem to be that Harvey had radically misunderstood Nardi's argument because of a fundamental ambiguity in Latin. In Latin the word *semen* means either semen or seed. The same ambiguity was once present in English, where 'seed' was used to mean semen, as in the biblical Onan spilling his seed upon the ground. Even modern scholars can get confused by this ambiguity: there's a striking example in an article published in *Medical History* in 1977. Nardi had compared the mysterious plague agent to invisible *seeds*, while Harvey had read him as comparing it to invisible *semen*. Outside the body semen rapidly loses its efficacy. It cannot be transported from one place to another or lie dormant. You don't get pregnant by touching someone else's clothes. Harvey, preoccupied with generation and so with semen, has completely missed the point of Nardi's argument. We know Harvey never received a reply from Nardi; we do not know if his letter ever reached him.

Nardi, as it happens, does not mention Fracastoro. His authority (apart from Lucretius himself) is Felix Platter. Platter, in his *De Febribus* (1597) and his *Quaestiones* (1625), had explicitly rejected arguments for the spontaneous generation of plague and syphilis, since these could not account for the fact that these were new diseases—if they could be spontaneously generated they would have arisen over and over again. The only explanation, Platter argued, is that these two diseases had come into existence once and once only—with the creation of the world—but that their distribution was erratic in time and space because they were spread by contagion. He thus carefully propounds the theory that these diseases are spread by seeds or germs; in the case of plague he notes that everyone agrees that external causes (miasmas) are also relevant; and he is prepared to accept, after a long debate with himself, that internal causes, the balance of the humours, are also relevant to susceptibility—though he recognizes that the fact that the plague strikes young and old alike might be taken to mean that the internal state of the body is as irrelevant as it is to someone being shot at by arrows. In any case, the germs themselves are a *sine qua non*, an essential prerequisite, a necessary condition for the spread of the disease. Platter is thus a proper germ theorist, the earliest known to me: in the case of contagious diseases, he denies that they can be spontaneously generated, and all his language implies that he is thinking in terms of animate contagion.

I never expected to come across Felix Platter. He does not appear

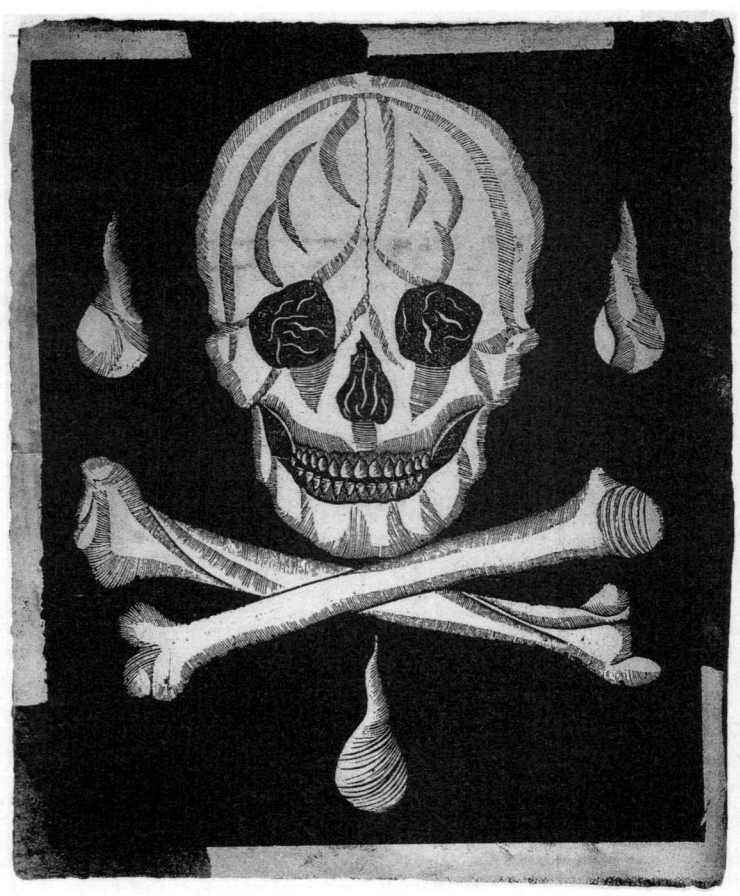

23. This seventeenth-century French woodcut of a skull and crossbones is believed to have been produced to be stuck up on the houses of people dying of plague. It reflects the belief that plague was contagious, and that it was therefore essential to avoid contact with people suffering from it.

in the literature (at least the English-language literature) on germ theory. I did not expect to find a proper germ theorist before the invention of the microscope. Yet he is hardly well-concealed. Harvey led me to Nardi, Nardi led me to Platter. If no one else has followed this route, it can only be because the intellectual origins of modern medicine remain a relatively unexplored field.

We might think that Leeuwenhoek, having discovered the *infusoria*, would immediately have decided that they were a possible cause of disease. Towards the end of his life he was certainly aware that some thought that plague is caused by little animals transported through the air. In 1702 he recognized that living beings could function like seeds: he discovered that the minute rotifer could be reanimated after years of dessication. But Leeuwenhoek never showed any interest in theories of animate contagion. Amongst his contemporaries, the only microscopist to develop such an argument was Nicolas Andry de Boisregard, whose *An Account of the Breeding of Worms in Human Bodies* (French 1700; English 1701) maintained that almost all diseases were parasitic infections: 'If we consider . . . the almost infinite number of little animals which microscopes discover to us, we shall easily find that there is nothing in nature into which the seed of insects may not insinuate itself, and that a great quantity of them may enter into the body of a man, as well as into those of other animals, by means of the air and aliments.'

The important point is not that Leeuwenhoek failed to develop this line of argument; it is that it is a line of argument that anyone could have developed who was familiar with Leeuwenhoek's work and with the idea of animate contagion: Leeuwenhoek's friend Nicolaas Hartsoeker, for example, who wreathed himself in tobacco smoke to kill off the invisible wormlets that carried the plague. There was no need to wait more than a hundred and fifty years for Lister, any more than there was any need to wait a hundred and fifty years for von Baer. From 1546 to the early 1720s there was a lively intellectual tradition debating animate contagion. Yet, as Charles and Dorothea Singer say in their study of this subject, 'from the year 1725 nothing of real value appeared on the subject' until the 1830s. Here too time stood still. Bonomo's work on scabies was not followed up until well into the nineteenth century. Agostino Bassi, a pupil of Spallanzani's, was the first to identify a 'germ' that was the cause of a disease: in 1835 he published work showing that the muscardine disease of silkworms was caused by a fungal infection—the work had been done years before, but he had lost time trying to find someone who was prepared to buy information about silkworm disease as a valuable commercial secret. His study of silkworms was followed by a series of publications, beginning in 1844, arguing that human diseases were caused by microscopic parasites. Bassi's research provided the model for J. L. Schoenlein's demonstration in 1839 that ringworm in humans was a fungal infection—the first occasion on which a human disease had been shown to be caused by a germ.

Between Bonomo's work and that of Bassi and Schoenlein a century and a half had been wasted because there was no interest in using the microscope to study disease. During this period obvious lines of enquiry were not followed up. Let me give one example, which is to be found in a little book published in 1810, and frequently reprinted thereafter. Charles Nicolas Appert's *L'Art de conserver, pendant plusieurs années, toutes les substances animales et végétales* is a practical manual on preserving food by bottling. Bottling and canning seem to us such elementary processes that it comes as a shock to realize that they are Appert's invention. Before him, food could be salted or dried, it could be preserved in brine, or vinegar, or syrup—these were all processes that transformed texture and taste. Appert's method was simple. You place food (a beef stew, say) in a glass container or bottle, and seal it with a very tightly fitting, fine quality cork, ensuring that no external air can reach it. (You needn't worry if there is some air inside the bottle.) You heat it over a prolonged period. And there you are—your food will last indefinitely. It has, we might now say, been pasteurized (though proper pasteurization employs lower temperatures than those used by Appert, and thus has less effect on the taste of the preserved food). But Appert is writing half a century before pasteurization, in a world in which everyone accepts that putrefaction is caused by exposure to air.

His method, he tells us, is opposed by many overeducated people who have assured him it is simply impossible. Against them Appert argued, as opponents of Spallanzani had done with regard to his work on spontaneous generation (which also involved heating food in sealed jars), that the method worked because heat transformed the air trapped in the bottles. In this respect Appert's preserves were just Spallanzani experiments, repeated over and over: the only difference is that Appert was preoccupied with eliminating putrefaction, Spallanzani with eliminating spontaneous generation. Neither recognized that the two enterprises are one and the same.

On p. xix of Appert's book you will find a report by a special commission established by the Society for Fostering the Nation's Industries to enquire into his methods. The head of the commission chose to use italics to emphasize one passage in his report:

> *What will appear even more extraordinary is that this same [bottled] milk, contained in a half-pint bottle, which had been opened a month ago so that part of it could be poured off, and then casually recorked, has been preserved almost without any alteration . . . I present it here in the same bottle, so that you can convince yourself of a fact that I would have had difficulty in believing, if it had been reported to me before I saw it with my own eyes.*

The italics are fully justified. According to all the established theories, once fresh air entered the bottle, putrefaction should immediately have followed. And yet sometimes it does not.

Why not? Fifty years later, Pasteur would show that everything depends on where you open the bottle. If it is in a room where the air is relatively free of germs, then putrefaction need not follow. But to understand this, you need to have grasped that micro-organisms cause putrefaction. Spallanzani claimed to be able to produce germ-free environments in which micro-organisms did not develop. But he had to break open his flasks in order to search inside them for micro-organisms. He kept them for days, but not for months or years. And so he never recognized what would seem to us an obvious fact: where there are no micro-organisms there is no putrefaction.

The first person to properly understand this was Schwann in 1837. He had shown that yeast was alive, and could be killed by heat, thus halting fermentation. Putrefaction, he set out to show, was also caused by micro-organisms, and could be halted by heating. What Spallanzani had not understood was that micro-organisms transform the world in which they live. Watching them through his microscope, Spallanzani saw them moving about in a world he had created. It never occurred to him that they had the power to transform their own world. Schwann, who had measured the transformation of sugar and starch into alcohol, understood this very clearly. The principle was later to be stated by Lister: 'We know that it is one of the chief peculiarities of living structures that they possess extraordinary powers of effecting chemical changes in materials in their vicinity, out of all proportion to their energy as mere chemical compounds.' Spallanzani did not know this, which is why he did not make the link between micro-organisms and putrefaction, and did not invent pasteurization.

Anyone who understood what Appert was doing when he bottled beef stew—killing germs—was in a position to invent antiseptic surgery, which is another way of applying the principle that germs cause putrefaction. Anyone familiar with Spallanzani's work should have been able to understand that Appert was killing germs and consequently they should have understood that, in the absence of micro-organisms, putrefaction will not occur. The passage in italics on p. xix of Appert's book was absolutely crucial evidence against the established theory of putrefaction and in favour of a germ theory of putrefaction, but nobody grasped its significance at the time. The fact that nobody did understand the significance of Appert's method of conservation does not mean that no one could have understood it. At any time after 1810 the germ theory of putrefaction and antiseptic surgery were real intellectual possibilities, even though the first appeared only in 1837 and the second only in 1865.

We have thus looked at three areas where research in the 1830s effectively took up from debates in the 1680s: reproduction, spontaneous generation, and animate contagion. I have discussed the last two topics as if they can be kept separate, but in reality they are intimately related. The idea of animate contagion only becomes powerful when it is combined with the denial of spontaneous generation, for then if one can kill the creatures that cause contagion one can eliminate disease. It is clear that a number of those who advocated animate contagion (e.g. Kircher and Hauptmann) were perfectly comfortable with the idea of spontaneous generation; others, such as Cogrossi, took it for granted that micro-organisms were never spontaneously generated.

One might think, then, that the question of spontaneous generation had to be resolved before germ theory could triumph. It comes as a surprise to discover that germ theory triumphed while the issue of spontaneous generation was still subject to a lively debate. The whole question was only finally resolved in 1877, when John Tyndall showed that the outcome of experiments on sealed and heated environments, or on heated environments containing only filtered air, depended not on the honesty and good faith, or technical competence and skill, of the experimenter, but on where he happened to conduct the experiment. Certain sorts of germ associated with hay could survive almost any amount of boiling, and, if hay had been in the room, could contaminate an experiment that was not supposed to involve hay at all. In 1876 Tyndall had made the mistake of introducing hay into his laboratory: thereafter, every spontaneous generation experiment he performed failed. To disprove spontaneous generation yet again Tyndall had to find a way of killing off these germs, which he showed was possible, not by prolonged boiling (which they survived unscathed), but by repeatedly heating them for short periods of time and then cooling them.

Since Tyndall, and only since Tyndall, spontaneous generation experiments can be made to work reliably—but Pasteur and Lister had already brought about a revolution in medicine by claiming (mistakenly, as it happens) that spontaneous generation had already been disproved. Two things made Pasteur's triumph possible, apart from the brilliance with which he devised and performed his experiments. The first was the enunciation of a new theoretical principle: *omnis cellula e cellula*—every cell comes from a cell—by Rudolf Virchow in 1858 (though the same idea had been expressed in different words by Robert Remak in 1852). This principle made spontaneous generation an impossibility. The second is the publication of Darwin's *Origin of Species* in 1859, for Darwin's arguments required that life had originated from non-life, and the debate over Darwinism thus turned into a debate over spontaneous generation. Pasteur turned almost immediately to work on spontaneous generation, and his arguments quickly won support because spontaneous generation now seemed tied to atheism and (by implication) political radicalism. Ironically,

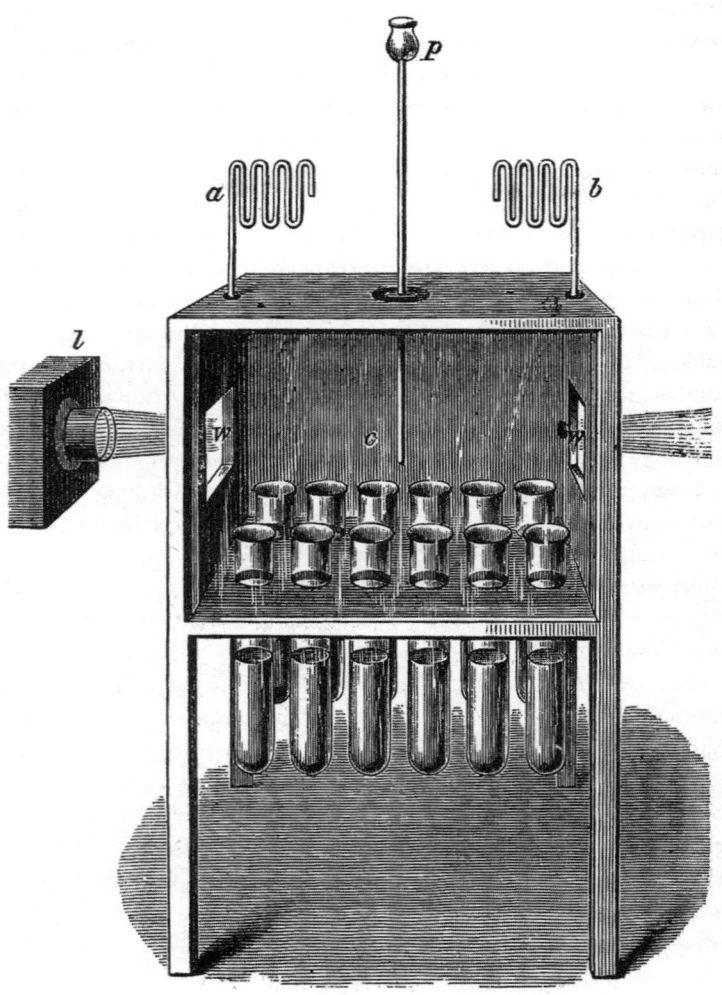

24. The apparatus devised by Tyndall for carrying out spontaneous generation experiments. The test tubes are exposed only to filtered air. The light
source shows that the air in the box contains no particles that reflect light,
and thus that it is sterile.

Tyndall was a Darwinist, but what his experiments seemed to show was that Pasteur was right, you cannot make life, at least in a test tube.

The debate on reproduction thus stood still for over a century. In some cases, such as the identification of the mammalian egg, obvious lines of enquiry were not followed up. In others, such as the inheritance of characteristics from the male, obvious objections went unanswered. In the parallel debate on spontaneous generation, similar experiments seemed to produce very different results, yet no progress was made towards explaining why this should be so. And arguments about animate contagion made no progress between Cogrossi in 1714 and Bassi in 1835. Why did biological knowledge remain so stable, why did it change so little between 1690 and 1830? It is no coincidence that this is precisely the period in which the microscope was out of fashion. Few scientists were working with microscopes, and most of those that were worked with ineffective compound microscopes. But, as we have seen, the microscope had gone out of fashion because there was no money in it. It would seem obvious that Leeuwenhoek's work on the grain weevil and the grain moth, and Malpighi's work on the silkworm, was intended to have practical application. So why was the microscope increasingly dismissed as a tool for serious research?

The answer is that the medical profession had set its face against the new research, and others followed where they led. In England, Willis and Lower abandoned their researches in 1669. Their one successor was John Mayow, who continued to 1675. Lower went on to become London's most fashionable doctor, but not because of his research record. In the nineteenth century no one could understand why the research of Boyle, Hooke, Willis, Lower and Mayow had been abandoned. In Holland the same thing happens to the work of Swammerdam and Leeuwenhoek. Here too the medical profession turned its back on the new research. Leeuwenhoek's hostility to doctors was such that the first thing he wanted to know when he was elected a Fellow of the Royal Society in 1680 was whether this meant that he could claim precedence over them. Swammerdam was qualified as a doctor, but never practised. Antonius de Heide, who also carried out important research with the microscope, was a practising doctor, until he repudiated the profession, denouncing medicine as murder. Steno, Van Horne and de Graaf had no successors. In France, not a single person who did significant research in biology in the course of the eighteenth century was a practising doctor or a teacher of anatomy. In the seventeenth century, Descartes had promised that sound natural philosophy would lead to a new medicine that would enormously extend life expectancy; by the end of the century even French Cartesian doctors had reconciled themselves to traditional medicine. Throughout Europe most people doing what we would now call biological research were amateurs. Science and medicine had parted company, above all because the doctors were determined that no scientific discovery would alter their traditional therapies of bleeding, purging, and vomiting.

In Rome, Giorgio Baglivi in 1699 called for a return to Hippocrates. In Amsterdam, in 1715, Johann-Conrad Barchusen denounced 'rationalist' medicine. In Angers, in 1718, Hunauld dismissed research into the causes of disease as a waste of time. These were the men teaching the next generation of doctors, and the claims they were making were already uncontentious. The key battles had already been fought. In 1683, in England, Gideon Harvey attacked 'those that flea [*i.e. flay*] dogs and cats, dry, roast, bake, parboil, steep in vinegar, limewater, or aqua fortis livers, lungs, kidneys, calves' brains, or any other entrail, and afterwards gaze on little particles of them through a microscope'. The doctor and philosopher John Locke, who was amongst the first to see *infusoria* in England (he had laughed at the very idea of such creatures until he saw them with his own eyes), and who, when in exile in Holland, had visited Leeuwenhoek and been shown the spermatozoa of a dog, remained loyal to his teacher, Thomas Sydenham, who held that theoretical research was irrelevant to therapy. Locke, in his *Essay Concerning Human Understanding* (1689), the most influential work of philosophy for eighteenth-century scientists, insisted that if we had microscopes for eyes, the knowledge we gained would be useless, just as someone who could see the inside of a clock but not its face would be unable to tell the time. God, in fact, has adapted our senses to our needs. Consequently, microscopical science is 'lost labour'. This was to restate Galen's view that the physician's hand is (thanks to God's careful design) the perfect instrument with which to measure hot and cold, dry and wet; now the physician's eyes too were perfectly adapted to their task.

In the same year, 1689, Paolo Mini, a former student of Marcello Malpighi at Bologna, mounted a direct attack on his professor: 'it is our firm opinion that the anatomy of the exceedingly small, internal conformation of the viscera, which has been extolled in these very times [*i.e. by Malpighi*] is of use to no physician'. Similarly, comparative research on insects and plants 'will not advance the art of curing the sick'. And again in that year, Girolamo Sbaraglia published a sustained attack on Malpighi's research with the microscope as contributing nothing to practical therapy. Malpighi spent the last years of his life composing a reply to his critics, and in that reply he made a decisive concession: microanatomy, he admitted, belonged to natural philosophy not medicine. There was no need for it to be taught in medical schools. Abandoned by the doctors, microscopy was everywhere on the defensive, and was to remain so for over a century and a half, until it re-entered the medical schools. Oliver Wendell Holmes (the Boston doctor and poet who was the father of the famous jurist of the same name) studied in Paris in the 1820s under the leading physicians of the day. 'I never saw a compound microscope during my years of study in Paris,' he wrote later; 'I never heard it alluded to by either professors or students.' Only in 1855, with Pasteur's revolution in full swing, was Rudolf Virchow able to announce that 'the promotion of microscopical research, initially mocked, is now victorious, and the language and concepts of pathological anatomy, indeed anatomy in general, are based in cellular pathology'.

Had microscopic research been actively pursued after the 1690s, traditional medical knowledge, and traditional medical therapies, would have been under threat. Medicine had integrated the discoveries of the dissectionists and vivisectionists into medical education; but the doctors refused to admit the relevance of the discoveries of the microscopists. By turning their back on the microscope they made it possible for traditional medicine to survive for a century and a half longer than it would have done had Leeuwenhoek's discoveries been taken seriously.

The opponents of the microscope did their job so successfully that even now the place of microscopy in the history of medicine goes largely unrecognized. Have I placed too much emphasis upon it? Bonomo, Cogrossi, Spallanzani, Bassi, Schwann, Pasteur, and Lister were all microscopists. At almost every step on the road towards the modern germ theory of disease we find the microscope—the important exception, whom we will come to later, is John Snow. It is no exaggeration to say that without the microscope doctors would never have acquired the capacity to defer death. Who would doubt that the telescope brought about a revolution in astronomy? Yet the equivalent claim, that the microscope brought about a revolution in the life sciences, including medicine, seems peculiar for a very simple reason, and one which we have been exploring: the revolution in medicine came almost one hundred and fifty years after the discovery of the microscope. Nevertheless the two were intimately connected, and the revolution would have occurred far earlier had Leeuwenhoek or Spallanzani had the pupils they deserved.

CONCLUSION TO PART II:
TRUST NOT THE PHYSICIAN

For centuries many people had understood that the claims doctors made on behalf of their therapies were exaggerated: we have seen that the first Hippocratics had to defend medicine against attack. In later centuries Christian critics would quote Mark 5: 25–7, on 'a certain woman, who had an issue of blood twelve years. And had suffered many things of many physicians, and had spent all she had and was nothing bettered but rather grew worse.' In early seventeenth-century England, plays are full of complaints about doctors. In Shakespeare's *Timon of Athens*, Timon says 'Trust not the physician; / His antidotes are poisons and he slays . . .' In Thomas Dekker's *The Honest Whore* we are told that it is far safer to fight a duel than to consult a doctor. In Ben Jonson's *Volpone* doctors are said to be more dangerous than the diseases they treat, for 'they flay a man / before they kill him'. Queen Elizabeth I would have agreed: she consistently refused to let the doctors treat her, even when dying. Half a century later the same complaints are to be heard in France, in Molière's *Le Médecin malgré lui* (1667) and *Le Malade imaginaire* (1673).

But the high point of anti-medical agitation was in England during the Interregnum, 1649–60. Nicholas Culpeper, publishing an unauthorized translation of the official medical *Pharmacopoeia* in 1649, asked

> Would it not pity a man to see whole estates wasted in Physick ('all a man hath spent upon physicians'), both body and soul consumed upon outlandish rubbish? . . . Is it handsome and well-beseeming a commonwealth to see a doctor ride in state, in plush with a footcloth, and not a grain of wit [*knowledge*], but what was in print before he was born? Send for them into a Visited House [*i.e. a house whose inhabitants have the plague*], they will answer they dare not come. How many honest poor souls have been so cast away will be known when the Lord shall come

to make Inquisition for Blood. Send for them to a poor man's house, who is not able to give them their fee, then they will not come, and the poor creature for whom Christ died must forfeit his life for want of money.

For all his complaints that doctors failed to treat the sick, Culpeper doubted the efficacy of traditional medicine (he favoured a mixture of herbs, of chemical remedies, and of astrology). The goal of his publications was to destroy the medical profession's monopoly of knowledge, so that if people wanted conventional therapies then they could employ them without recourse to doctors. For it was obvious to everyone that doctors had a financial interest in claiming to be the only ones able to cure diseases, just as lawyers had a financial interest in seeing disputes reach the courts.

In 1651, Noah Biggs said it was impossible not to be aware of 'the cruelties and unsuccessfulness of the medical profession'. George Starkey, in 1657, complained that doctors engaged in 'bloody cruelty . . . tormenting the patient'. Some of the people who saw that medicine was not what it claimed to be were themselves doctors. Biggs was convinced that even doctors were aware of 'their own unsuccessfulness'. Take the example of Antonio Durazzini, who practised in the small town of Figline near Florence. From there he reported to the government of Florence in 1622 on an epidemic of a deadly fever. He had been treating those who could afford it, treating them with bloodletting and other traditional remedies, but he noted in his official report that 'more of those who are able to seek medical advice and treatment die than of the poor', who of course received no treatment. Here was a simple test of the effectiveness of medicine, but Durazzini may not have been able (or willing) to recognize it as such. Perhaps he thought the poor were peculiarly robust.

There is no such ambiguity about the views of Latanzio Magiotti, a contemporary of Durazzini's and doctor to the court of the grand duke of Florence. Count Lorenzo Magalotti tells us that

> our dear friend Magiotti said quite openly [*that doctors and medicine were useless*] and when Grand Duke Ferdinand asked how in all honesty he could accept money from patients knowing he could not cure them he replied: 'Most Serene Highness, I take the money not for my services

as a doctor but as a guard, to prevent some young man who believes everything he reads in books from coming along and stuffing something down the patients which kills them.'

Similar examples could be found in every age and society, at least where the records are good enough to record indiscreet conversations and private doubts. 'Therapeutic nihilism', the belief that most conventional medical therapies did not work, became the norm amongst sophisticated (particularly Parisian) doctors in the 1840s as a result of a new interest in statistics. In 1860, Oliver Wendell Holmes, who had received a Parisian medical education, expressed a good deal of sympathy for the view that 'on the whole, more harm than good is done by medication'. But a scattering of therapeutic nihilists is to be found in every age and place. As long as therapies were not subject to statistical tests, however, such sceptics had limited influence.

There had always been important disputes amongst doctors themselves about which therapies were most effective. For example, there were disagreements about which diseases were best treated with bleeding, how much blood should be taken, where it should be taken from, and how it should be taken (by lancet, cup, or leech). These disagreements were recurrent and unresolvable within conventional medicine, and sometimes they amounted to an attack on significant aspects of that medicine. We have already seen that Girolamo Fracastoro in 1546 insisted that many diseases were contagious. Because he no longer saw such diseases as the result of unbalanced humours, he naturally also went on to question the utility of bloodletting as a therapy when dealing with such diseases. Over time, his arguments won ground: by the 1630s a significant minority amongst Italian doctors thought that letting the blood of plague victims did more harm than good, and they seem to have been a clear majority by the end of the century. The Dutch physician Ysbrand van Diemerbroeck, whose work was translated into English in 1666, expressed similar views that were widely influential. In 1696 a work by Dominicus La Scala entitled *Phlebotomia Damnata*, or bloodletting condemned, provoked a rapid response entitled *Phlebotomia Liberata*, or bloodletting set free.

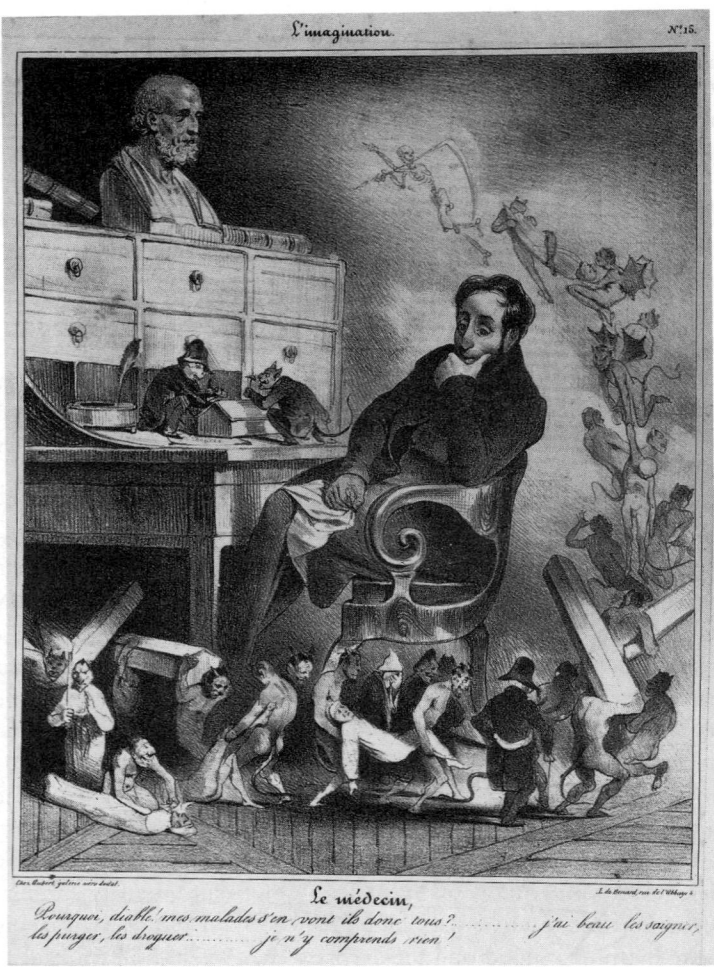

25. This lithograph by Honoré Daumier, which appeared in 1833 shows a doctor (sitting under a bust of Hippocrates) asking himself 'Why the devil do all my patients go off like this [i.e. in coffins] . . . I do my best by bleeding them, purging them, drugging them . . . I just don't understand it!' It marks the moment when doctors began to recognize that conventional Hippocratic remedies were ineffective.

Fracastoro and Diemerbroeck did not deny that there was an appropriate use of traditional Hippocratic remedies, but sustained attacks on the whole Hippocratic tradition of treatment by contraries came from Theophratus Paracelsus (d. 1541) and Jan Baptiste van Helmont (d. 1644). They held that diseases never resulted from imbalances of humours. Rather each disease was a specific condition, it had an 'essential thingliness', it was a 'lively, active thing', and must therefore be treated with specific remedies. God had so designed the world that there were remedies for every disease if one only knew where to look for them. Their arguments were taken up by the religious radicals of mid-seventeenth-century England who, as a consequence, did not hesitate to question the efficacy of traditional therapies.

Why were these disputes never resolved by practical trials? Doctors relied instead on what we would now call anecdotal evidence: individual case histories of successful treatment. They continued to do so long after the unquestionable authority of the ancients had been destroyed, first by Vesalius and then by Harvey. Real tests only began in the 1820s. Once they began, medicine was inevitably thrown into a prolonged crisis, a crisis that peaked in the 1850s when the core therapy of bloodletting was shown to be ineffectual. That crisis was only resolved by the triumph of germ theory in the years after 1865. But the triumph of germ theory was itself only the result of a major shift towards microscopy (which reassumes prominence in the 1830s) and towards laboratory research, a shift that had taken place at least thirty years earlier.

Historians often puzzle over why that shift occurred, and why there was extensive investment in laboratories when at first the results were mediocre. At least part of the answer lies in the urgent need, first apparent in the 1820s, to find an effective form of medical therapy as traditional therapies began to be exposed as worthless. The laboratory did not bring about the demise of conventional medicine; rather the demise of conventional medicine led to investment in the laboratory. Germ theory did not supplant Hippocratic medicine and its therapies; rather the demise of Hippocratic medicine was a precondition for the triumph of germ theory.

Medicine, until the 1820s, was rather like a religion, in that its claims were not subject to practical testing. For some 2,350 years doctors relied on a series of therapies—bleeding, vomiting, purging—which did not work and actually did harm. These therapies, of course, looked as if they were doing good. They mobilized the placebo effect, and moreover, in the case of bloodletting they resulted in what appeared to be immediate (if not lasting) benefit: a slower pulse, a reduction in temperature and inflammation, a sound sleep. Faith in these apparent benefits, however, would not have survived any comparative trial.

The real puzzle with regard to the history of medicine before germ theory, as with the history of astrology, is working out why medicine once passed for knowledge. The case of medicine is, at first sight, rather more intractable than that of astrology, for it is hard to disprove astrology: one would need to compare the lives of a group of people all born at the same moment. In the absence of such a test, it is easy for astrologers to claim their arguments fit the facts. But medicine, it would seem, is quite different, for it is obvious how to set about testing the efficacy of a medical therapy. All that is needed is to take a group of patients with similar symptoms and treat some of them and not others. Moreover, it would seem, it is hard to tell when an astrologer is right and when wrong; but in the case of medicine there is a convenient crude measure of success to hand: the ratio of those patients who are still above ground to those who are now below ground. If it is this easy to put medicine to the test, why did traditional medicine survive untested into the nineteenth century?

There are three good reasons for medicine's unique status as a mythical technology. First, doctors were trying to achieve outcomes that the body's natural healing processes were also working to achieve. It was easy to assume that if a patient recovered, then the therapy they had received was responsible, though in 1657 George Starkey had claimed that only a third of diseases were cured, but less than a tenth were cured by the doctors. He was trying to expose the illusory character of medical success. The first study of the body's capacity to heal itself, however, did not appear until 1835: the American Jacob Bigelow's *Discourse on Self-Limited Diseases*. By 1860, when

Oliver Wendell Holmes set out to analyse the profession's 'tendency to self-delusion', the fallacy of much traditional medical reasoning was apparent to almost everyone. Second, the placebo effect meant that an ineffectual intervention could often result in a cure. This reinforced the illusion of success, and for a very long time the working of the placebo effect was entirely invisible both to doctors and to their critics. Its discovery in 1800 marks the moment at which it first became possible to begin to assess the true effectiveness of medical intervention. It is this discovery, which we will explore in the next chapter, not the new anatomy, which marks the beginning of the end for Hippocratic medicine. Third, in order to test a therapy you need to have a concept of a disease as being not a disorderly condition of a particular patient, but a typical condition of many patients, for only then can you be confident that you are comparing like with like. In order to think of diseases in these terms you needed to have either a concept of contagion, or a concept of epidemics such as was developed by Sydenham.

These three obstacles made it difficult to recognize that medicine did not work. In addition, there was (or appeared to be) a fundamental ethical obstacle to the carrying out of the most simple of comparative tests. Doctors were supposed to do the best for their patients. They had no right to withhold treatment, if a treatment was available, and no right to try out an untested remedy when a reputable therapy existed. But this ethical dilemma existed in appearance, not reality. Early modern doctors only treated those who could afford to pay for them. Vast numbers of people went without treatment, so that there would never have been any shortage of people to use as a control group had anyone wanted to compare the effects of treatment with no treatment.

Much more constraining was the tacit obligation to give the minority who could afford to pay orthodox treatment. 'I will abstain from harming or wronging any man', says the Hippocratic oath. From the beginning this must have been understood as meaning 'I will do what other supposedly competent doctors would do in these circumstances.' Underlying the apparent ethical obstacle was a pressure to conform that made it impossible to test new therapies against old ones. In 1663 Robert Boyle told a story that became popular of a doctor who had refused to try alternative remedies, saying of his patient 'briskly . . . "Let him die if he will, so [long as] he die *Secundum Artem*"', i.e. while receiving orthodox treatment.

Such an attitude was commonplace. In 1818, Alexander MacLean, a Scottish doctor working in India, was busy recommending swallowing mercury as a therapy for almost all diseases. His opponents pointed out that too many of his patients died; he replied that this was because he treated only the most desperate cases. He proposed a randomized trial to compare his treatment with bloodletting. His opponents refused, saying one should not experiment with the lives of men, 'as if', said MacLean, 'the practice of medicine, in its conjectural state, were anything else than a continued series of experiments upon the lives of our fellow creatures'. MacLean was quite right about that, if not about mercury. The efficacy of bloodletting was completely untested; nevertheless, it was universally employed. For as the Helmontian Noah Biggs had complained in 1651, the theories of the Hippocratic doctors were quite irrelevant, 'nothing but trifles and anxious disputes'. What really mattered were their basic remedies, especially purging and bloodletting. These were 'the slender hinges' upon which 'the whole huge bulk of the art of healing seems nowadays to be moved'.

These reasons—the illusion of success, the placebo effect, the tendency to think about patients not diseases, the pressure to conform —go some way to explaining why medical therapies continued to be employed that were at best ineffectual, and more often than not positively harmful. But do they go far enough? The missing element, it might be thought, is formal regulation. Once medicine became, in the thirteenth century, a profession licensed by the universities of Europe, and by governments who took for granted the value of medical degrees, Hippocratic doctors were not competing on equal terms with the various unofficial suppliers of therapy, and the efficacy of Hippocratic medicine was (except for brief moments, such as the English Civil War and the French Revolution) already officially predetermined and beyond question. Official medicine, it might be claimed, went unquestioned because doctors were legally authorized

in roughly the same way that theologians were. The validity of orthodox medicine was established by the decrees of university, state, and
church, and was thus not open to question. The test of truth within
the scholastic intellectual world of the universities was intellectual
coherence, not practical effectiveness, and as long as medicine met
that test it was subject to no other. Medicine was (in the world of the
universities, if not always outside) a monopoly, and because it was a
monopoly there was no need for it to prove its superiority by comparing alternative therapies.

An interesting test case is provided by Gianna Pomata's *Contracting
a Cure* (1998). Pomata's book is a study of a panel of doctors, the
protomedicato, in early modern Bologna that adjudicated on complaints by patients that they had not received good value from those
they had paid for treatment. She set out, she tells us, intending to
write a history of how popular healers had been marginalized and
outlawed by the medical profession; but she was so captivated by the
voices of the patients in the judicial records that she turned aside to
write a history of the sick persons' experience of their illness and
treatment, and in particular of the working of a system where patients
were entitled (or at least believed they were entitled) to withhold
payment or reclaim their money if they had been treated without
being cured.

Pomata constantly stresses that doctors and legal authorities
contested the right of patients to refunds where there was no cure, but
she argues that at the beginning of the seventeenth century this right
was recognized by the court of the *protomedicato* if there was a prior
agreement that payment should be by results, while by the eighteenth
century it was consistently being rejected. You have to read her book
with some care to discover that she does not identify a single example
of a patient successfully enforcing an agreement for a cure against
a licensed and qualified doctor. We are told that at the end of the
sixteenth century 'the protomedici endorsed the terms set by the
agreements for a cure, including the principle of payment for results',
but this turns out to be true only in the case of claims against barber-
surgeons; for qualified doctors it was already the case that 'for the
patients, a therapeutic transaction was fair if the healer respected the

terms of the cure agreement; for the protomedici, it was fair if the practitioner medicated according to the official rules'. As far as doctors were concerned the agreement for a cure had already ceased to exist when the *protomedici* were established in 1581. Doctors were prepared to reduce the fees claimed by other doctors in practising orthodox medicine when those fees were exorbitant or when patients were impoverished, but they were not prepared to rule that the failure of the therapy meant that they were not entitled to payment. Not only were the sentences of the tribunal in malpractice cases 'always favourable to the practitioners', but in disputes over whether doctors were entitled to payment when they had failed to cure the tribunal consistently ruled in favour of the doctors.

In Bologna doctors did not have a monopoly: they practised alongside, and in competition with, other licensed healers, including barber-surgeons and apothecaries. But they practised on terms that were biased in their favour, for it was they who sat on the tribunal which decided if healers were entitled to payment and if there had been malpractice. Elsewhere, though, doctors did not have even this degree of control over the marketplace for therapy. In England, effective regulation of the medical profession broke down in the course of the seventeenth century. In eighteenth-century America there was something close to a free market in medical training, different therapies competed against each other without hindrance, and regulation only became the norm late in the nineteenth century. If we go back to ancient Greece and Rome, then competing schools of medicine had confronted each other on equal terms. Hippocratic medicine did not depend on regulation to establish itself, and it did not collapse when regulation collapsed.

So it is one thing to harbour doubts, and quite another to put those doubts to a test. It is one thing for the efficacy of traditional medicine to be questioned, another thing for its efficacy to be tested. We need to add a further factor to the illusion of success, the placebo effect, the tendency to think about patients not diseases, and the pressure to conform, and that factor is the absence of statistical thinking. Statistical thinking does not come naturally. You can tell if a building is properly designed by seeing whether it stands or falls. You can see if a clock tells time by comparing it with a sundial. But making a comparison between two competing therapies is a quite different enterprise. It requires a statistical comparison of two sample populations.

Sophisticated statistical thinking was born along with probability thinking in the 1660s. It was soon being used to predict life expectancies using the London 'bills of mortality' (first analysed by John Graunt in 1662) which showed the ages of all those who died in London. But for a hundred years life insurance continued to be sold, like a lottery ticket, at the same price for everyone, which meant that the young paid far too much for it and the old paid far too little. Statistical thinking was slow to develop and there was considerable resistance to it. Until that resistance had been overcome, there could be no trial of traditional medical therapies. As we shall see, that resistance has never been entirely overcome, and arguments from statistics are given much less prominence in histories of medicine than they ought to be. It is the combination of these five factors—the illusion of success, the placebo effect, the tendency to think of patients not diseases, the pressure to conform, the resistance to statistics—which explains, if anything can, the intolerable delay in testing the efficacy of orthodox medicine.

At this point we need to ask what sort of historical explanation we hope to find. Do we want to prove that there was never any possibility of testing orthodox medicine before the 1820s? We would be wrong. Do we want to prove that the obstacles to testing orthodox medicine were great, but not insuperable, before the 1820s? Then we would be right, but an argument of this sort cannot absolve all those doctors who practised an ineffectual form of therapy from some responsibility. If we provide too strong an explanation of why traditional medicine was not put to the test until the nineteenth century, then we will inevitably lose sight of the fact that plenty of people could see that it didn't work. It is difficult to strike the right balance here, but the resilience of orthodox medicine is far more significant than the persistent criticism it encountered. The stress needs to fall on medicine's appearance of success, and on the ease with which it saw off competition from Paracelsians and Helmontians.

III. MODERN MEDICINE

8
COUNTING

In the eighteenth century, serious thought about the impact of medical intervention concentrated on one question: the merits of inoculation against smallpox. The procedure was simple: a thread covered with pus from a fresh pock on someone mildly infected with smallpox was pressed into a cut on an arm and on a leg of someone who had not yet had the disease. This usually resulted in a very mild case of smallpox, from which the individual rapidly recovered, and remained henceforth immune against further attacks. Smallpox inoculation had been practised in Turkey, China, and elsewhere, but was first publicized in Northern Europe by Lady Mary Wortley Montagu, who had lived in Constantinople (and who herself was seriously disfigured by smallpox). She persuaded the princess of Wales to have two of her daughters inoculated in 1722. A trial was first made on six condemned prisoners in Newgate, on the understanding that if they survived they would be released. All six survived. As a result inoculation became increasingly widespread thereafter.

Inoculation against smallpox raises a number of delicate questions and, although it is easy for us to assume we know what the right answers to those questions were, contemporaries were right to find them difficult and perplexing. At one level the argument was straightforward. The chances of dying from inoculated smallpox were at first estimated at one in a hundred—in 1723 James Jurin, who was Secretary to the Royal Society, and thus in a position to correspond with experts around the world, did a careful study which produced a figure of one in ninety-one. The chances of dying from normal smallpox were known to be around one in ten (excluding those who died under the age of 2). Most people were exposed to smallpox at some point. It therefore seemed to follow straightforwardly that inoculation

154   MODERN MEDICINE

would save large numbers of lives. John Arbuthnot, a mathematician and doctor, published in 1722 a statistical analysis that showed that one in twelve deaths in London were due to smallpox, though he still preferred the claim that smallpox killed one in ten of the susceptible population on the grounds that many infants cheated smallpox by dying before it had a chance to infect them. (This line of argument was mistaken: Haygarth and Percival would later show that one quarter of all smallpox fatalities were children under one year in age, and Arbuthnot had probably underestimated the proportion of Londoners dying of smallpox.) Similar but more complex calculations by James Jurin resulted in a more reliable figure of one in seven. Inoculation, it was argued, would save 1,500 lives a year in London alone. In England, despite a few vocal objectors, the case for inoculation was generally found persuasive.

In France, on the other hand, inoculation was rejected by the medical establishment, particularly the Paris Faculty of Medicine—which continued to reject Harvey's theory of the circulation of the blood, along with one of the few effective drugs to be discovered in the Renaissance, cinchona, from which quinine (for the treatment of malaria) was later to be extracted. French doctors did not practise inoculation, and those in France who wanted to be inoculated had to turn either to laymen or to foreign doctors. Nevertheless, French intellectuals, such as Voltaire and La Condamine, urged their compatriots to copy the English. In 1760 La Condamine's friend Maupertuis persuaded the great Swiss mathematician Daniel Bernoulli to enter the debate. Bernoulli set out to calculate the increase in average life expectancy that would result from inoculation, and came up with the figure of two years.

In reply Jean d'Alembert questioned whether most people were actually prepared to run a significant risk (say one in a hundred) of immediate death in order to gain only two years. The state and the society might gain if everyone was inoculated, but d'Alembert had considerable sympathy with cowardly individuals who had no desire to put their lives at risk by a deliberate act. He saw himself as taking the viewpoint of a mother of a small child rather than a father. You could not reduce, d'Alembert argued, the sort of decision involved in deciding to be inoculated to a simple cost–benefit analysis. There was no simple ratio that would allow one to weigh an increased life expectancy against a risk of immediate death.

In the 1750s inoculation techniques in England were greatly improved, the infected matter now being introduced under the skin rather than into the bloodstream. The procedure was safer. The practice of first bleeding and purging people before inoculation, and of subjecting them to a special diet and a period of rest lasting for a month prior to the operation, in order to ensure they were fighting fit, was abandoned. Inoculation thus became cheaper, and consequently more widespread.

But a person inoculated against smallpox was capable of giving the disease in its virulent form to anyone they contacted. Early calculations of the number of lives that might be saved by inoculation made no attempt to factor in the number of people who might be infected as a result of inoculation. While smallpox was endemic in large cities such as London, and almost everyone was exposed to it sooner or later, it was epidemic in smaller towns and villages. In Chester, for example, one person died of smallpox in 1773, but 202 died (more than one third of all deaths) in 1774. In small towns and villages some people may have escaped exposure throughout their lifetimes. To inoculate a few people in such a town or village would be to endanger all the others. In a small village or even town this problem could be avoided by inoculating everyone at once, but in a large city this was not feasible. Thomas Dimsdale, who had been paid £10,000 to inoculate the empress of Russia, and who had carried out a general inoculation of the whole population of Hertford, argued in 1776 that there had been a recent increase in deaths from smallpox in London, and that indiscriminate inoculation was responsible. He thought that the recently founded (London) Society for the General Inoculation of the Poor, which made no attempt to quarantine those it had inoculated, was recklessly endangering lives. John Haygarth agreed.

Haygarth was acutely conscious of the problem of contagion: he was the first to stress the importance of isolating patients with fevers from others in order to halt the spread of infections. He first advocated the establishment of separate fever hospitals, but then became convinced that it was easier to manage infections than he had supposed—that one needed, for example, to come within eighteen inches of a smallpox sufferer in the open air to become infected. So he became convinced that separate wards were all that was required.

Dimsdale and Haygarth, however, had very different responses to the possibility that inoculation might save the lives of a few but at the same time spread the infection to many others. Dimsdale was prepared to abandon the poor of London to the natural course of the infection. Haygarth wanted a national campaign to eradicate smallpox entirely, but the basis of such a campaign had to be the effective isolation of the newly inoculated. What was crucial to Haygarth's grandiose project of 1793 was that he had made a close study of how smallpox actually spread. He had established the length of the infective period. He knew how close you had to be to someone to be infected even if he did not know why (smallpox is spread by droplets —he thought it was disseminated by a poison or *virus* dissolved in the air). Haygarth knew that the disease was normally transmitted between people who were close to each other, but that it did not require physical contact. He had thus been able to draw up Rules of Prevention that were tested out in Chester between 1778 and 1783 and were shown to halt the spread of the disease. The Rules banned anyone who had not had smallpox from visiting anyone who had the disease, or anyone who had the disease from leaving their house until the scabs had dropped off, and even then not before their body and their clothes had been washed. Anything the patient had touched was to be washed, and anyone dealing with the patient must wash their hands before touching anything that was to leave the patient's house. The Chester experiment immediately became the model for inoculation campaigns in larger cities such as Leeds and Liverpool. Ideally the Rules were to be enforced by a mixture of carrot and stick— monetary rewards for those who complied, and fines for those who did not (even today in the UK, doctors receive a financial reward for meeting inoculation targets). Applied on a national scale they would, Haygarth was well aware, require an army of government inspectors. But he was convinced that only if one combined inoculation with the Rules could one be confident that one was making progress towards eliminating the disease rather than helping to spread the infection. Haygarth called on another brilliant mathematician, John Dawson, to calculate the impact of his proposals: according to Dawson, they would result in the population of Great Britain being increased by a million within fifty years (a claim which is roughly compatible with Bernoulli's calculated gain in life expectancy).

This whole argument became irrelevant within a few years. Jenner's cowpox vaccination (1796) provided immunity to smallpox, but cowpox was not itself contagious amongst humans. Vaccination, unlike inoculation, carried with it no risk of spreading smallpox.

It is easy to tell the story of inoculation as if it was clear from the beginning who was right and who was wrong. Lady Mary Wortley Montagu, Voltaire, Arbuthnot, Bernoulli are the heroes of this story and the Paris Faculty of Medicine the villains. If you tell the story this way Dimsdale's concerns have to be belittled, as they were by some contemporaries. There was always some fluctuation in death rates from smallpox, even in London where they were more stable than elsewhere, so that Dimsdale's evidence for a rising death rate in the years 1768 to 1775 (which he attributed to more widespread inoculation) was and still is dismissed. In modern accounts, inoculation becomes indistinguishable from vaccination, an obvious benefit to mankind.

But this way of telling the story ignores the fact that early campaigners for inoculation gave no thought at all to the risk of spreading the disease. Dimsdale and Haygarth were the first to recognize the possibility of what we now call iatrogenesis, to see that one had to measure the adverse consequences of medical intervention as well as the benefits. (The word *iatrogenic* dates to 1924, but at first it seems to have been used only in the context of mental diseases exacerbated by psychiatrists; the earliest example the *OED* gives of its use in the context of a disease that is not psychological in origin dates to 1970.) Those who practised inoculation before the formulation of Haygarth's Rules were relying on blind faith. They knew that smallpox was contagious, but they did not want to consider the possibility of contagion. Bernoulli felt sure that he could show that society benefited from inoculation, even if no mathematical formula could determine if individuals did—but his confidence was spurious. Without proper study of the period of infectivity and the mode of transmission the consequences of inoculation were unpredictable and incalculable. The caution of those such as the Paris Faculty of Medicine who feared that inoculation might do more harm than good was entirely sensible.

Haygarth's achievement in formulating his Rules represents an important moment in the history of medicine, for Haygarth was the first to identify and seek to minimize the unintended consequences of medical intervention. In fully recognizing the risks as well as the rewards associated with inoculation, and in taking the risks as seriously as the rewards, Haygarth provided a model of how medical knowledge and public health policy should progress. But in the textbooks the risks associated with inoculation disappear from the story, and as a consequence Haygarth either disappears from view or becomes an uncritical advocate of inoculation. As we shall see, the Rules are not the only reason why Haygarth deserves to be better known.

In sixteenth-century Venice novel therapies were sometimes tested on condemned criminals—there could, it seemed, be no objection to experimenting with the life of someone who was already about to die. We have seen a similar trial of smallpox inoculation was conducted in London in 1721. But such tests did not compare two groups of patients. Early examples of printed accounts of such trials include those described by Ambroise Paré in his *Oeuvres* of 1575. Paré was a great surgeon, the first to tie off blood vessels during amputations, although unfortunately he did not see the need to apply a tourniquet, which meant that fatalities were still frequent. He describes two occasions (in 1537–8) when he carried out a comparative trial of two therapies.

At stake was the conventional view that bullets did not only tear a hole in you, and gunpowder did not just supply an explosive force: gunpowder, it was held, killed by poisoning as well as burning, and gunpowder residue on bullets introduced poison into the body, and so an anti-venom remedy (oil of elderberry, to which a little theriac had been added, producing a paste usually applied boiling hot) should be administered. On one occasion Paré was called to deal with a drunk who had accidentally set fire to his flask of gunpowder, which had exploded in his face. Following the advice he had earlier received from an old woman on how to treat burns from boiling oil, he applied an ointment of onions to one side of his patient's face, but the usual remedy to the other: the onion ointment clearly prevented the blistering and scarring which disfigured the side of the face to which the burning paste had been applied. On another occasion Paré ran out of the paste while treating a group of soldiers who had been hit by gunfire, so that some were treated only with a cold dressing of egg yolk, turpentine, and oil of roses, which was normally applied only as a second dressing, after the burning paste, to encourage healing. These patients did far better than those who had received the orthodox treatment, which Paré abandoned thereafter. Paré's publication in 1545 of a treatise on how to treat gunshot wounds served to kill off the myth that gunpowder acted as a poison.

Paré had no doubt that he had learnt something important from his two comparative trials, yet he never conducted any others. Surgery was a relatively empirical and untheoretical discipline, and surgeons were not doctors—they had not benefited from a university education, which is why in England they are still titled 'Mr'. Surgeons like Paré were therefore relatively open to innovation. It is also important that gunpowder burns and gunshot wounds were new to Western medical science. Guns had only been important on the battlefield for a hundred years or so. Paré did not have to question long-established authority in order to abandon theriac. No one was being asked to deny the authority of Hippocrates or Galen.

Paré's trials were accidental and *ad hoc*. We have to wait more than a hundred years for a proper clinical trial to be proposed. In *Oriatrike*, Johannes Baptista van Helmont (d. 1644), not himself a doctor and, as we have seen, a bitter opponent of conventional medicine, suggested that five hundred sick people should be randomly divided into two groups, one to be treated with bloodletting and other conventional remedies, and the other by his alternative therapies. Helmont was not nearly influential enough to bring such a trial about, but his followers continued to propose such tests of the efficacy of his remedies. Thus in 1675, Mary Trye claimed that if her medicine for curing smallpox was tested against the conventional remedy of bloodletting, then it would be found that the proportion of her patients that survived would be twice that amongst those receiving conventional therapies. In 1752 the philosopher and doctor of divinity (but again, no doctor) George Berkeley suggested a similar experiment to test the value of tar water in the treatment of smallpox. These are lonely examples that show that there was nothing particularly difficult about conceiving of a clinical trial. But none of these proposals came from doctors, and actual trials never took place. Had such trials been performed, they might have shown either that the therapies favoured by the Helmontians and by Berkeley were better than the standard bleeding and purging, or possibly, like the mercury therapy favoured by MacLean in 1818, even worse.

One doctor has become established in the literature as the inventor of the modern clinical trial. James Lind was a Scot, and he qualified first as a surgeon and then as a doctor. In 1753 he published *A Treatise of the Scurvy*. Scurvy is a condition that we now know is caused by vitamin C deficiency. The first symptoms are swollen gums and tooth loss. The victim soon becomes incapable of work. Death follows, though not swiftly. The standard medical therapies were (of course) bleeding, and drinking salt water to induce vomiting. A patent remedy was Ward's Drop and Pill, a purgative and diuretic. In other words, scurvy was understood in humoral terms and the remedies were the conventional ones—bleeding, purging, and emetics.

Scurvy becomes a problem only if you have a diet that contains no fresh vegetables. In the Middle Ages castle garrisons subjected to prolonged sieges came down with it, but it became a major problem only with the beginning of transoceanic voyages: if you are healthy to begin with, you will only show symptoms of scurvy after you have been deprived of vitamin C for some ten weeks. Ancient and medieval ships stayed close to land and came ashore regularly to take on water and fresh food; but once ships embarked on long ocean voyages they needed to carry food supplies which would not perish, usually salted beef and hard tack (dried biscuit, notoriously full of weevils). Any fresh vegetables were hastily consumed before they could perish.

One estimate is that two million sailors died of scurvy between Columbus's discovery of America and the replacement of sailing ships by steam ships in the mid-nineteenth century. This estimate is much too high. Typhus killed more sailors than did scurvy, and sailors who disappear from ships' crew lists have often deserted rather than died. So while it has been claimed that of 184,899 sailors who served in the British fleet during the Seven Years War, 133,708 died from disease, mostly scurvy, the real figure may be closer to one tenth that, of which the majority will have died of typhus. It has been argued that almost 90% of the 2,000 men commanded by Anson on a voyage to the Pacific in 1740 died, nearly all of scurvy; but the death rate was 70% (largely from typhus and shipwreck), and most of those with scurvy survived. The normal death rate from scurvy on long voyages was not, as has been claimed, 50%: 5% would be nearer the mark. Still even if only 100,000 died of scurvy between 1500 and 1850, the medical profession were responsible for almost all these deaths (for, when good arguments are beaten from the field by bad ones, those who do the driving must bear the responsibility).

In 1601 Sir James Lancaster had stocked his ship, sailing to the East Indies, with lemon juice. The practice became standard on ships of both the Dutch and English East India Companies in the early seventeenth century. The power of lemons to prevent scurvy was known to the Portuguese, the Spanish, and the first American colonists. By the early seventeenth century the problem of scurvy had effectively been solved. Yet this treatment made no sense to doctors with a university education, who were convinced that this disease, like every other, must be caused by bad air or an imbalance of the humours, and it was under their influence (there can be no other explanation) that ships stopped carrying lemons. This is a remarkable example of something that ought never to occur, and is difficult to understand when it does. Ships' captains had an effective way of preventing scurvy, but the doctors and the ships' surgeons persuaded the captains that they did not know what they were doing, and that the doctors and surgeons (who were quite incapable of preventing scurvy) knew better. Bad knowledge drove out good. We can actually see this happening. There is no letter from a ship's surgeon to his captain telling him to leave the lemons on the dock, but we do know that the Admiralty formally asked the College of Physicians for advice on how to combat scurvy. In 1740 they recommended elixir of vitriol (dilute sulphuric acid), which is completely ineffectual, but now became standard issue on navy ships. In 1753 Ward's Drop and Pill also became standard issue.

Historians, far from holding doctors responsible for the one hundred thousand or so deaths from scurvy, credit a doctor with discovering the cure. James Lind was a surgeon (and not yet a qualified doctor) aboard HMS *Salisbury* in 1747, serving in the Channel Fleet. Of his crew of 800, 10 per cent were suffering from scurvy. Of the eighty, he took twelve and put them all on the same diet. He divided the twelve into six pairs. Two were given cider each day; two were given elixir of vitriol; two were given vinegar; two were given salt water; two were given a herbal paste and a laxative; two were given oranges and lemons. Some other sailors were given nothing. Within a week those on oranges and lemons were cured (and the ship's stock was exhausted, so the remedy could not be tried on others). Those on cider made some slight progress. The rest deteriorated. Lind had conducted the first clinical trial since Paré; indeed he was the first medical doctor to conduct a clinical trial. He had discovered an effective therapy; eventually that therapy was universally adopted. The modern history of therapeutics begins here.

Or does it? Lind waited six years, and first qualified as a doctor, before publishing his remedy. His book, *A Treatise of the Scurvy*, was four hundred pages long, and only four pages were devoted to his clinical trial. The rest were devoted to a complex theoretical argument and to a review of the literature. His basic theory was humoral, although he presented a modernized humoralism in that he stressed the importance of perspiration through the skin for the overall balance of the humours. (Sanctorius, in the early seventeenth century, had been the first to try to measure the amount of fluid lost through perspiration.) The cause of scurvy, Lind argued, was a blockage of the pores caused by damp air. Lemons, he claimed, had a particular capacity to cut through this blockage: he thought this was something to do with their being acidic, although he admitted that other acids (such as vinegar) lacked the requisite quality. Contemporary readers saw nothing decisive in Lind's arguments, and one can think of some obvious objections to them. Did sailors not sweat? If the problem was an imbalance of the humours, why should traditional remedies not work? The book was translated and reprinted, but it did not alter the practice of ships' surgeons.

In 1758 Lind was appointed chief medical officer at the Royal Naval Hospital at Haslar, the largest hospital in England. There he was responsible for the treatment of thousands of patients suffering from scurvy. But he treated them with concentrated lemon juice (called 'rob'), and he concentrated the lemon juice by heating it to a temperature close to boiling. He also recommended bottled goose-berries. In both cases, the heat destroyed much of the vitamin C, and Lind conducted no tests to compare his concentrates with fresh fruits. As a result he seems to have gradually lost faith in his own remedy, which had actually become less effective, and he became increasingly reliant on bloodletting. When he published in 1753 he reported the views of the Polish doctor Johan Bachstrom, who main-tained that scurvy 'is solely owing to a total abstinence from fresh vegetable food and greens, which is alone the true primary cause of the disease.' But in 1772, in the 3rd edition, he added a postcript insisting one could not reduce the cause of scurvy to a matter of diet. Lemons were often effective, but scurvy 'may be cured by medicines of very different and opposite qualities to each other, and to that of lemons.'

Thus Lind himself had no clear understanding of exactly what it was that he had discovered in 1747, and no grasp of the importance of the clinical trial as a procedure. He conducted various trials of therap-ies at Haslar, not only on methods for treating scurvy, but also on drugs to alleviate fever: he reported in his *Essay on Diseases Incidental to Europeans in Hot Climates* (1771), that he had 'conducted several com-parative trials, in similar cases of patients.' But what he gave his readers were conventional case histories, and it seems that none of his later trials, despite all his efforts, produced significant results—pre-sumably because he was always trying one ineffective remedy against another. Moreover his therapeutic practice remained entirely conventional. We find him on a single day bleeding ten patients with scurvy, a woman in labour two hours before her delivery, a teenage lunatic, three people with rheumatism, and someone with an obstruction of the liver. He was cautious when bleeding people with major fevers, but only because he preferred to use opium or to induce vomiting. If Lind had invented the clinical trial, then he had done a profoundly unsatisfactory job of it.

Why then has Lind become a major figure in the history of medicine? The answer is that when the formalized clinical trial for new drug therapies was introduced in the middle years of the twentieth century there was a natural desire to look back and find its origins. In 1951 A. Bradford Hill published his classic article 'The Clinical Trial' in the *British Medical Bulletin*. It contains references to nine scientific publications, all in the previous three years. It was often assumed at the time that the clinical trial was a brand new invention, introduced to test the latest drugs. Streptomycin had been discovered in 1944, and in 1946 the (British) Medical Research Council began testing it on patients with tuberculosis—the results were published in 1948. Because streptomycin was in short supply it was decided that it was ethical and fair to choose by drawing lots which patients would receive the drug and which serve as controls. This was not, as the *British Medical Journal* claimed at the time, the first randomized clinical trial; but it was the moment when the role of the controlled trial won general recognition. It was precisely at this point that Lind was rediscovered to help give the clinical trial an appropriate history, with an article by R.E. Hughes on Lind's 'experimental approach' in 1951, and an article by A.P. Meiklejohn in 1954 on 'The Curious Obscurity of Dr James Lind.'

If Lind did not succeed in curing scurvy, who did? In 1769 Captain James Cook's *Endeavour* set sail on the first great voyage of exploration in the Pacific. When it returned more than two and a half years later, not one of the crew had died from scurvy. Cook had primarily relied on sauerkraut to keep the scurvy at bay, and in fact it does contain a little vitamin C. He had also taken on fresh vegetables whenever he made landfall. On his next voyage, which lasted seven years, he took a number of remedies—Lind's concentrated lemon juice, an infusion of malt called 'wort', carrot marmalade, and soda water amongst them. Taken together the remedies worked, and though Cook thought soda water useless, and never administered the carrot marmalade, he had no idea which of the others were effective and which were not. Cook at one point acknowledged that a careful inspection of the ship's surgeon's journal might clarify the point; but no such inspection was ever made. On his third voyage, in search of the Northwest Passage, Cook was killed in Hawaii (1779); but his crew returned after a voyage of four and a half years without having lost anyone to scurvy. Cook had shown that long voyages could be undertaken without crews suffering from scurvy, but no one knew exactly how he had achieved this; he did not know himself. The consensus view however, supported by appropriately elaborate medical theories, was that it was the wort that had done the trick; when a merchant sea captain wrote to the Admiralty in 1786 informing them that lemon juice mixed with brandy always cured scurvy he was told straightforwardly that he was wrong:

> trials have been made of the efficacy of the acid of lemons [i.e. rob] in the prevention and cure of scurvy on board several different ships which made voyages round the globe at different times, the surgeons of which all agree in saying the rob of lemons and oranges were of no service, either in the prevention or cure of that disease.

The first person in the navy, after Lind, to give unconditional support to lemon juice was Gilbert Blane, appointed physician to the West Indies Fleet in 1780. Blane seems first to have established the peculiar efficacy of lemons by trial and error, for he started with both lemons and wort on board his ships. In 1793 a formal trial of lemon juice was made, at Blane's suggestion, on the *Suffolk*: the ship was at sea for twenty-three weeks, crossing from England to the East Indies, without taking on fresh food. Lemon juice was administered preventatively, and when scurvy appeared the dose was increased, with satisfactory results. In 1795 lemon juice became part of the daily ration throughout the navy, so that by the end of the 1790s scurvy had been virtually eliminated. It had taken fifty years for Lind's discovery of the curative power of lemon juice to be generally adopted, and no further controlled clinical trials had been conducted. It was Gilbert Blane, not Lind, who had persuaded the navy to adopt lemons, and the triumph of lemon juice over wort had done nothing to further the idea that therapies should be subjected to systematic comparative testing. Blane had never conducted a comparative test of lemon juice against other therapies.

Lind's failure to press home the implications of his single trial, and his failure to repeat it successfully, mean that he actually deserves to be left in obscurity. If one wants to identify key figures in the invention of the clinical trial it would be better to look elsewhere. In 1779, for example, Edward Alanson published *Practical Observations on Amputation*. He recommended new techniques—the cutting of a flap to close the wound, and the laying together of wound edges to facilitate healing. He compared his results before he adopted his new methods (10 fatalities out of 46 amputations) with his recent results (no fatalities out of 35 amputations). This persuasive statistical argument had a major impact on surgical technique in England and Europe (though the French remained sceptical). Alanson's control group was historical, and he did not randomly select who was to receive what treatment; but he was using numbers to effect. In 1785 William Withering published a careful account of his use of the foxglove (the active ingredient being digitalis) to treat a total of 163 patients suffering from dropsy (or what we might now diagnose as congestive heart failure). But in practice digitalis, once it had established itself in the pharmacopoeia, was soon being used to treat a whole host of diseases, and was often not used to treat dropsy—bad knowledge had once again driven out good.

Even more important than the work of Alanson and Withering is John Haygarth's *Of the Imagination as a Cause and as a Cure of Disorders of the Body* (1800). Haygarth wanted to debunk the claims made on behalf of some instruments, metal pointers called 'tractors', presumably because they were used to 'draw out' diseases, that had been patented by an American, Elisha Perkins (1741–99), and that were sold at the astonishing price of 5 guineas. These briefly had an enormous success, particularly in the fashionable and moneyed world of Bath, where Haygarth had retired from the practice of medicine. He set out to show that he could obtain remarkable cures, first of rheumatism and then of other conditions, with pointers that vaguely resembled those of Perkins, but were made of any other substance. What made the cure, he argued, were not the patented tractors, but the demeanour of the doctor and the credulity of the patient. The fact that fake (or as he quaintly called them 'fictitious') tractors worked as well as real ones did not only show that the real ones had no peculiar therapeutic quality. It also proved 'to a degree which has never been suspected, what powerful influence upon diseases is produced by mere imagination'. This was the discovery of the placebo effect: the word placebo was already in use in English in 1772, although Haygarth does not use it himself.

One of Haygarth's colleagues had also elucidated the limits of the imagination in effecting a cure. He had used Haygarth's fictitious tractors on a woman who suffered from pain in her arm and from an inability to move her elbow joint, which had become locked by an abnormal growth of bone. Her imagination had cured her of her pain, and she thought it had given her new movement in her elbow; but in fact if one watched closely one could see her elbow was still locked, and she was merely compensating more successfully with increased movement in her shoulder and wrist.

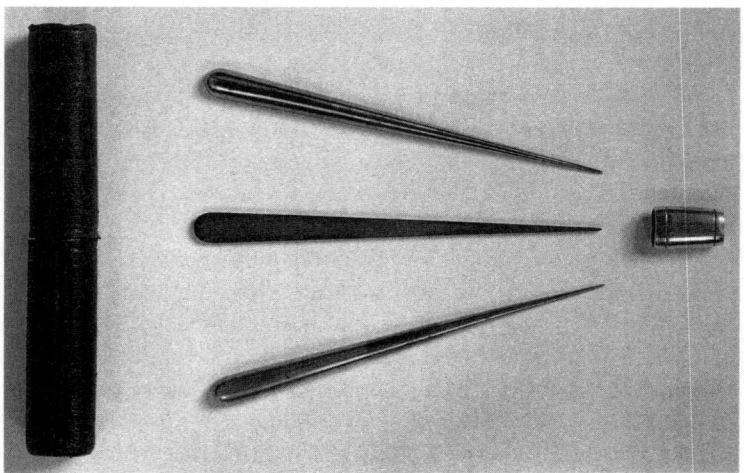

26. A set of Perkins tractors.

Haygarth also noticed a small number of cases in which patients got worse not better when the fictitious tractors were applied: thus he showed that imagination could cause as well as cure diseases. In such cases, we might say, the symptoms Haygarth was producing in his patients were psychosomatic in origin; but Haygarth did not pursue this line of thinking. More importantly, he did not reverse it: he did not claim that the symptoms that were cured by fictitious tractors were psychosomatic. This is important because doctors had known since ancient times that emotions could give rise to physical symptoms and that these symptoms could be cured by a change in the patient's emotional state. Edward Jorden in 1603, for example, had discussed the case of a young man who had fallen out with his father and then fallen victim to 'the falling sickness' (epilepsy): he had been cured by a kind letter from his father. Haygarth did not argue that the fictitious tractors only worked to cure conditions that were psychological in origin.

Haygarth believed that his experiments with fictitious tractors explained why a famous doctor was often more successful in his practice than someone without an established reputation, and why a new medicine was often more successful when it was first introduced than when it had been around for some time. One doctor or one medicine might be more successful than another because they were more effective in eliciting the cooperation of the patient's imagination. For real success, he claimed, it was important that both the doctor and the patient should be believers: 'Medical practitioners of good understanding, but of various dispositions of mind, feel different degrees of scepticism in the remedies they employ. One who possesses, with discernment, the largest portion of medical faith, will be undoubtedly of greatest benefit to his patients.'

Here Haygarth's conclusion was at odds with his own research. He had successfully shown that sceptics, using fictitious tractors, could, by pretending to believe, elicit results indistinguishable from those achieved by true believers using genuine Perkins tractors. His doctors had cynically used the patter employed by the advocates of the Perkins tractor, without believing for a moment what they were saying. Why pretend otherwise? One can only assume that Haygarth wanted to protect himself against the charge of encouraging lying and hypocrisy when he asserted, against the evidence of his own trials, that if one wants to touch one's patient's heart one must speak what one feels.

But what Haygarth had done was suggest that much standard medicine relied entirely on the placebo effect. Within a few years the arguments he had deployed to explain the apparent success of Perkins tractors were to be employed by his medical colleagues to explain the success of homeopathy. Oliver Wendell Holmes's essay on 'Homeopathy and its Kindred Delusions' (1842) contains an extended discussion both of the Perkins tractors and of Haygarth's fictitious tractors. But the genie was out of the bottle. If the placebo effect could explain the success of Perkins tractors and of homeopathy, what part of orthodox medicine was based on a similar delusion? Haygarth's importance lies in the fact that he was the first to ask this question.

Haygarth does not appear in histories of medicine for his discovery of either iatrogenesis or the placebo effect. They make no mention of Perkins tractors. For them Haygarth is important (if at all) as an advocate of smallpox inoculation. Instead of discussing Haygarth on the power of the imagination, they discuss the commission established by the king of France in 1785 to enquire into the cures achieved by Franz Anton Mesmer. Mesmer had achieved enormous success in Paris by claiming that diseases could be cured by manipulating the patient's 'animal magnetism', a process that induced trances, fits, and faints. The commission, which reported in 1785, included the great chemist Lavoisier, Benjamin Franklin, and the now infamous Dr Joseph Guillotin. The commissioners set out to subject Mesmer's claims to tests very similar to those that Haygarth was to devise a few years later to test the Perkins tractor. Thus they had someone trained by Mesmer 'mesmerize' a glass of water, and then they offered a patient five glasses of water to drink, including amongst them the mesmerized glass. The patient fainted on drinking from one of the glasses—but it was a glass of ordinary water. They concluded that Mesmer's cures were produced by the power of his patients' imaginations, and their enquiry certainly was one of the first systematic attempts to devise a 'blind' test of a therapy: as such it is an important moment in the birth of evidence-based medicine. But, unlike Haygarth, the royal commission did not go on to acknowledge that the power of the imagination must play a role in orthodox medicine; they failed to recognize that what we would now call the placebo effect is present in all medical treatment. They failed to direct their scepticism towards orthodox medical practice.

Medical historians would seem to have a similarly blinkered vision. They are interested in Haygarth because he discovered how to prevent infections spreading from one patient to another, and in the French royal commission because it pioneered the blind trial. Yet, as we have seen, what is really important about Haygarth is that he was the first properly to understand (if not to name) both iatrogenesis and the placebo effect: he understood that hospitals spread infections and that inoculation might spread smallpox; and he recognized that conventional medicine relied in large part on the same power of imagination as that evoked by the Perkins tractor.

The initial usage of the word *placebo* was to refer to a pill (made of flour, sugar, or some other inert substance) given to reassure a patient for whom no effective treatment was available. The first use of the placebo in clinical trials (a procedure which implies an understanding of the placebo effect) was apparently in Germany in 1834. There trials were being carried out to test the effectiveness of homeopathy. In these tests homeopathy was systematically compared with placebo therapy (pills made of charcoal), and found to be no more effective. This was the first occasion on which the test of effectiveness in a therapy was defined as being more effective than a placebo—one of the tests employed today (therapies can also be assessed against no treatment, or against alternative treatments).

By the early nineteenth century there was thus nothing problematic about the idea of a controlled trial of a medical therapy. In 1816 an Edinburgh military surgeon called Alexander Lesassier Hamilton described, in a thesis published though so obscure as to be little read (it was in Latin), a model trial that he had carried out on sick troops in 1809, during the Peninsula War. The troops were arbitrarily divided into three groups, one third receiving bloodletting and two-thirds not. Of the 244 soldiers treated by alternative methods six died, while of the 122 whose blood was let, 35 died. Unfortunately Lesassier Hamilton was an incorrigible liar who led a dissolute life (we know a great deal about him because all his private papers were seized during divorce proceedings, and were preserved for posterity in the archives of his wife's lawyers), and the story is almost certainly an invention. His detailed diary for 1809 contains no reference to any trial. Nevertheless, Lesassier Hamilton invented only to impress, so his story does tell us what he thought his examiners would want to read.

The most important advocate of the new numerical method was Pierre-Charles-Alexandre Louis, whose *Recherches sur les effets de la saignée* were first published in a learned journal in 1828, then expanded as a book in 1835. They were translated into English and published in America (1836). Looking back in 1882, Oliver Wendell Holmes, who had studied under Louis, thought this 'one of the most important written contributions to practical medicine, to the treatment of internal disease, of this century'. In his original article, Louis looked at three conditions, pleuropneumonia, erysipelas of the face, and angina tonsillaris, all classified at the time as inflammatory diseases, and therefore believed to respond well to bleeding. In the case of pleuropneumonia every patient (there were a total of 78) was bled, but some were bled sooner than others and some more frequently than others. Louis could find little indication that when or how often the patient was bled affected the outcome, whether one looked at the proportion who survived or, amongst the survivors, at the amount of time it took to recover to good health. In the case of erysipelas of the face Louis looked at thirty-three patients, twenty-one of whom were bled. Those who were bled recovered three-quarters of a day sooner than the others. In the case of angina tonsillaris Louis looked at twenty-three severe cases, of whom thirteen were bled. In the case of the patients who were bled, recovery took place a day and a quarter earlier than in the case of the patients who were not bled. The conclusion was obvious and even italicized: 'bloodletting, notwithstanding its influence is limited, *should not be neglected in inflammations which are severe and are seated in an important organ*'.

In the edition of 1835, Louis considered additional cases. Again, every case of pleuropneumonia, now called pneumonitis, had been bled. The conclusion was now rather different from before. It was 'that bloodletting has a happy effect on the progress of pneumonitis, that it shortens its duration; . . . that patients bled during the first four days recover, other things being equal, four or five days sooner than those bled at a later period'. (The 'four or five days' claim is very puzzling: on Louis's own figures, the difference was two-and-three-quarters days.) He then ended his book with a survey of recent books on bloodletting. The survey is wonderfully amusing, were the subject not so deadly serious. Here, for example, is a small part of his discussion of a doctor Vieusseux, who had published a treatise on bloodletting in 1805:

> Our author, as may easily be conceived, has not been very difficult as to particular examples; and in adducing proof of this I am embarrassed only as to a choice among the cases he states. Thus on the subject of abdominal diseases, which he thinks are often attended with gangrene, he says, 'I have seen an instance of the alternate use of venesection and leeches in a female thirty years of age, who was subject to pain in the abdomen, and who suffered two or three days without fever and without tenderness on pressure. Suddenly the pain became very violent, and was accompanied with fever and vomiting. She was bled eleven times, and meanwhile had leeches to the anus twice, in the course of seven or eight days; she recovered rapidly, escaping suppuration, which should be avoided at any cost.'
>
> Vieusseux considers this observation neither as short nor as incomplete; he gives it as if it were approved. Now I will ask the reader what is proved by an observation, relative to an abdominal affection, which contains no account of the form and volume of the abdomen, of the condition of the discharges, of the colour of the matter vomited, of the expression of the face, nor of the state of the pulse . . .

Louis's conclusion is 'that many authors consider facts only as a sort of luxury, to be used as seldom as possible'.

I have carefully outlined Louis's argument because extraordinary misconceptions appear in the books that discuss him. It is said that Louis had set out to show that bloodletting was pointless. Yet he clearly believes it to have some considerable merit and advocates it in the treatment of all the diseases he studies. One commentator claims Louis had shown bloodletting postponed recovery in cases of angina tonsillaris. Louis believed he had shown the opposite. There was nothing in Louis's book to persuade doctors to abandon venesection, and it is clear that he did not abandon it himself. On closer inspection it seems that Louis interpreted his data in a fashion that was strangely biased in favour of venesection. His own figures suggested early venesection shortened the disease by 2.75 days, yet he claimed that 'other things being equal' it shortened it by four or five days. In fact, he had shown that other things were not equal. Those bled early were on average eight years and five months younger than those bled late, which in itself is sufficient to explain their more rapid recovery. Again, it is said that Louis was concerned to criticize the contemporary use of leeches, which had been strongly advocated by François Broussais. It is true that he seems to have little time either for leeching or vessication (blistering or cupping). But it is quite clear that what he is trying to study is the merits of venesection, and that he believes the only way of establishing how far venesection helps is by comparing cases statistically.

Since Louis's conclusion was that bloodletting, though it never halted a disease in its tracks, was still good for patients, one is bound to look closely at his statistics. After all, if he was right, why do we not still let blood? Table 1 is a simplified version of his table detailing the second group of patients with pneumonitis, twenty-five of whom survived the disease. The top row shows the day on which blood was first let. Each cell below records the number of days it took a particular patient to recover, until the final row, which shows the average recovery time for patients in that column.

I have already suggested that Louis's argument that those bled early recover more quickly than those bled late is spurious, and that the form in which he presents his figures conceals a correlation between youth and rapid recovery. Table 2 gives the information he supplies reorganized in a way that it never occurred to him to organize it.

This suggests that, over the age of 20, the older you are the longer recovery takes. But it is also clear that these tables reflect a hopelessly

TABLE 1. Recovery times of Louis's second group of patients with pneumonitis

Day on which blood first let	2	3	4	5	6	7	14
Days to recovery	15	11	14	9	25	11	22
	16	27	19	28	21	19	
	11	28	14	11	12	18	
		9	12			24	
			13			21	
			15				
Average for column	14	18	14	16	19	18	22

TABLE 2. A reorganization of Louis's data, showing recovery time in days according to the age of patients

Age (rec. time)					
18 (9)	20 (9)	30 (16)	41 (28)	50 (14)	60 (11)
18 (18)	22 (19)	36 (15)	42 (13)	58 (21)	60 (21)
19 (27)	23 (19)		45 (14)	58 (22)	61 (15)
	24 (12)				61 (25)
	24 (11)				62 (24)
	25 (11)				66 (28)
	29 (11)				67 (12)
Average time 18	13.1	15.5	18.3	19	19.4

small sample. A few more cases bled early and slow to recover, or bled late and fast to recover, and Louis's results would be quite different. A few more teenagers who recovered rapidly, and my results would be quite different. Louis has no way of testing to see if the distribution of numbers in columns actually reflects an underlying pattern—a statistically significant correlation—or is purely random.

Louis, the great advocate of the statistical method, thus played fast and loose with his own statistics. Above all, his approach was hopelessly crude because he had no test of statistical significance. Louis faced plenty of contemporary critics who argued that medicine was an art not a science, and that each case had to be considered individually. He also met critics, such as the great Claude Bernard, who argued that science was concerned with causal connections, and that consequently 'statistics can never yield scientific truth'. What were needed were experiments conducted in the laboratory.

But Louis also faced the criticism of mathematicians. In 1840, Jules Gavarret published his *Principes généraux de statistique médicale*. There he argued that no results of the sort that Louis was claiming to produce would be reliable unless they were based on several hundred observations. Thus Louis had observed (in a book published in 1834) 140 cases of typhoid fever, with 52 deaths and 88 recoveries, and concluded that 37 per cent of patients recovered. Gavarret showed that with a sample this size the margin of error was roughly 11 per cent, so that all one could reliably say was that between 26 and 48 per cent of patients recovered.

In 1858, Gustav Radicke also set out to expose the fallacy in using small samples to draw large conclusions. He was particularly interested in samples where you measured something (e.g. days taken to recover) and he argued that it was very important in such cases to establish whether the measurements tended to be homogeneous or heterogeneous. If the measurements were homogeneous, a fairly small sample might produce a reliable result, but if they were heterogeneous (in the case of Table 2 above, recovery times vary between 9 and 27 days for teenagers, and between 11 and 28 days for people in their sixties) there was obviously a significant possibility that further measurements would alter the averages and transform the conclusions. He proposed a mathematical test to establish when a result derived from figures of this sort was, and when it was not, trustworthy.

Despite the efforts of Gavarret and Radicke to apply sophisticated probability theory to medical statistics, no nineteenth-century medical researcher made use of the methods they proposed. Nevertheless, as we shall see, statistics lay at the heart of the most important achievements of nineteenth-century medicine. In 1801 a reviewer of one of John Haygarth's books still felt it worth noting that 'the facts or cases upon which the whole of the reasoning . . . is founded are exhibited in the form of tables . . . This synoptical mode of recording and exhibiting cases in an inquiry of this sort is attended with many advantages.' We might go so far as to say that the statistical table was the first direct threat that Hippocratic medicine had faced in over two thousand years. By 1860 the revolution represented by the table was complete. 'Statistics have tabulated everything—population, growth, wealth, crime, disease', wrote Oliver Wendell Holmes. 'We have shaded maps showing the geographical distribution of larceny and suicide. Analysis and classification have been at work upon all tangible and visible objects.' Looking back towards the end of his life, in 1882, over the recent history of medicine, what impressed Holmes was not the rise of the laboratory, but the triumph of statistics: 'if there is anything on which the biological sciences have prided themselves in these latter years, it is the substitution of quantitative for qualitative formulae'. One of the greatest medical breakthroughs of the nineteenth century, John Snow's account of the transmission of cholera, was due to the careful use of statistics, and even of maps, but before we look further at the statisticians, we need to look at the alternative intellectual tradition that for a time promised to revolutionize medical knowledge, at experimental physiology.

9
BIRTH OF THE CLINIC

Modern medicine, medical historians generally (although I think mistakenly) agree, begins in France shortly after the French Revolution of 1789. The Revolution had completely disrupted medical education—for a short time no new doctors graduated (the university faculties of medicine were abolished in 1792), and at the same time anyone was permitted to practise medicine—but when order was restored in 1794 medical education, medical diagnosis, and medical research were placed upon a new footing. Education now required the presence of trainee doctors in hospital wards where they would follow the diagnosis and treatment of actual patients—this was not a new idea, for it can be traced back to Renaissance Florence, and was common in late seventeenth-century Holland, but it was now applied systematically for the first time. A medical education was now acquired on hospital wards, and not just in a university setting, in the lecture theatre and the dissecting room.

At the same time the nature of diagnosis changed. Until late eighteenth-century France, the standard medical encounter, the one that shaped the thinking of the profession, was one in which a fee-paying patient consulted a doctor of her own choice. In this exchange the patient always had the upper hand for the doctor could be dismissed at any time. As we have seen, the doctor usually did not examine the patient; commonly his curiosity was satisfied by feeling the pulse or inspecting the urine, both of which stood in as substitutes for the patient's actual body. The information the doctor relied on was primarily provided by the patient's own words. But in post-revolutionary France the standard medical encounter came to be seen (despite the fact that the majority of doctors were still seeing private patients in their homes) as one between a doctor who was paid for by the state and a patient who had no control over her own treatment, an encounter which took place in a hospital setting. Here, the power relations were reversed: a patient who misbehaved or did not follow the doctor's instructions would be sent home. There was central control over the distribution of patients: if a doctor was known to be working on a particular disease, suitable patients would be directed to see him. In these encounters, doctors paid less and less attention to what the patient said was the matter, and more and more attention to their own direct observation of the patient's body.

Underlying this was a more profound change. In the past doctors had sought to alleviate symptoms as described by the patient: what mattered was that the patient should feel better, if not immediately (most patients must have felt worse after repeated purging) then in the medium term; in the end the measure of success was a subjective one. But now, in the first decades of the nineteenth century, doctors were seeing patients in considerable numbers, and when these patients died (as a high proportion of them did) their bodies were routinely autopsied. One doctor working at La Charité hospital said that in the twelve years he had worked there he believed not a single patient who had died had escaped autopsy. What the doctor now sought to do was predict, on the basis of his inspection of the patient, what would show up at autopsy. The doctor's task was to read the symptoms he could perceive in the living as indicators of a hidden condition that would only be exposed to view in the dead. His project was to move in the mind's eye from the surface of the body to the interior, and soon very simple new tools—such as the stethoscope —were to be devised to make this task easier.

This task was complicated by the fact that the interior of the body was now being observed in a different way. In the past, autopsies had primarily been concerned to locate the cause of death in a particular organ, and each organ was seen as having a particular function within the body. But now each organ was seen as being constructed out of a number of different types of tissue (eventually twenty-one different types were identified), and the same types of tissue were found throughout the body, so that at autopsy it was seen that the same type of lesion, affecting the same type of tissue, could be found in very different organs. The founding text of this new anatomy was François-Xavier Bichat's *Traité des membranes*, of 1799, followed by his *Anatomie générale* of 1801: Bichat had arrived in Paris in 1794, at the age of 22, but he had been quick to impress, probably because he had begun learning medicine at an early age from his father, a professor of medicine at Montpellier. In Bichat's work the body was no longer described as a city made up of different buildings; instead it was seen as a city made up of different buildings constructed from a narrow range of materials, so that rotting wood might equally be found in a town hall, a country cottage, or a castle; just so an inflamed membrane might be found in lung, intestine, or eye-socket, or rather an inflamed membrane of a particular sort, for Bichat distinguished membranes into three distinct types.

This set of interlocking transformations—a new analysis of the body's components; a new observation of the patient's body; a new relationship between doctor and patient; a new medical education— was the subject of a famous book by Michel Foucault, *The Birth of the Clinic*, first published in French in 1963 and in English translation in 1973. The word 'clinic' might be better paraphrased as 'teaching hospital', though for Claude Bernard the clinic was not an institution but an enterprise, 'the study of a disease as complete as possible'.

Four important developments took place over a generation or two within this new medical world. First, doctors became slowly aware of the limits of their powers. When the young Oliver Wendell Holmes went to Paris for his medical training in the 1820s, there were still doctors around who would arrive on the wards in the morning and order that every patient, no matter what was wrong with them, should have their blood let. The fashionable theories in the 1820s were those of François Broussais: he thought diseases originated in inflammation, and the treatment for inflammation was bloodletting, though he favoured leeches rather than venesection. Slowly doctors were forced to recognize that their treatments seemed to do little good. In a hospital setting, where the patients were under constant supervision, they could scarcely blame the patients for failing to follow their instructions, so they came face to face with the limits of their own powers. Wendell Holmes went back to America from

France convinced that most therapies were useless—a view that scandalized American doctors, but fairly represented the most advanced French thinking. His hero was Louis, whose work we have already discussed. The clinic gave birth to what is sometimes called 'therapeutic nihilism'. And therapeutic nihilism was entirely justified. For the first time in more than two thousand years doctors were finally beginning to acknowledge that they did little good, and some harm.

Second, and more slowly, as statistics were collected and treatments compared, it became apparent that hospitals were actually very bad places in which to be ill. In Britain, Sir James Simpson, the discoverer of chloroform anaesthesia, established that 40 per cent of amputations performed in hospitals resulted in death; on the other hand only 10 per cent of amputations performed outside hospitals were fatal. Simpson memorably concluded: 'A man laid on an operating table in one of our surgical hospitals is exposed to more chances of death than was the English soldier on the field of Waterloo.' The hospital itself seemed to be a cause of disease, and Simpson coined the word 'hospitalism' to define the problem.

What was the cause of the problem? One answer was that hospitals were rather like slums: dirty (patients were often put into beds that had been occupied by other patients, with sheets covered in blood and pus), smelly (with the air pervaded by the smell of rotting flesh and gangrene), and crowded (with as many beds as possible squeezed into large wards). Often they were built near graveyards and industries. In terms of traditional thinking, both the analysis and the solution were straightforward: the problem was miasma, or bad air; the solution was ventilation and improved cleanliness. In the Crimean War it was found that wounded soldiers operated on in tents had a better chance of recovering than those operated on in hospitals: the very buildings themselves appeared to be at fault. Miasma must be countered with hygiene. Florence Nightingale was one of the great exponents of this line of argument—and improved hygiene did help. But cleanliness alone did not seem enough to prevent the spread of infection, and by the 1860s many were arguing that the big city hospital would have to be abolished, that patients would have to be treated at home or in little cottage hospitals. Within two generations the new medicine was in a profound crisis: its therapies didn't work, and its key institution, the hospital, was a death trap, a 'charnel house', as John Tyndall put it.

This new awareness of just how dangerous medical intervention could be is usefully marked by the coining in 1860 of the phrase *primum non nocere*, 'first do no harm'. The first person to use it was Thomas Inman, who claimed (mistakenly) to be quoting Thomas Sydenham. But the phrase was quickly picked up and attributed not to Sydenham but to Hippocrates—despite the fact that Hippocrates wrote in Greek, not Latin. In reality it is an invention of 1860 and its rapid attribution to Hippocrates represents the invention of a tradition. Newly aware of the extent to which doctors were capable of doing harm, the medical profession reassured themselves with the thought that Hippocrates had shared their concern.

At the same time as the hospital system destroyed itself from within, two new developments were taking place, the one an extension of the other, just as the identification of hospitalism was a natural extension of therapeutic pessimism. First, a small group of doctors, mainly in Paris, came to feel that medical knowledge would never be complete if it relied entirely on the inspection of patients and the dissection of cadavers. What was needed was the application to medicine of the experimental method, an enterprise that would make possible new developments in physiology. Since there were limits to the experiments that could be performed on humans the new science was to be based on animal experiments. Here again Bichat was a key figure. One of Bichat's concerns was to establish what actually happened when people died. Death, he realized, was not a uniform process. Sometimes the heart stopped first, and the other organs of the body then failed; at other times, for example if someone drowned, it was the lungs that first ceased to function, followed by unconsciousness and the stopping of the heart; or again an injury to the brain might be fatal, though the lungs and heart were in good order.

Bichat, the founder of the new account of human anatomy in terms of different types of tissue, devised experimental methods for studying the progress of death through the body. For example, one could model the failure of the lungs by passing venous blood rather than arterial blood into the heart to be pumped around the body. Bichat tried connecting the heart of one dog to the veins of another, but it was hard to get the pressure right and the blood flowing in the right direction. He had more success tying off the flow from the lungs and injecting venous blood in its place—brain death followed, as if from asphyxiation. These experiments were reported in *Recherches physiologiques sur la vie et la mort* (1800).

Experimental physiology meant that for the first time doctors needed a specialized space in which to conduct research. 'Every experimental science requires a laboratory', wrote Claude Bernard in his *Introduction to the Study of Experimental Medicine* (1865). Medicine followed the path pioneered by physics and chemistry in becoming a laboratory science. The first medical laboratories were straightforwardly places for conducting vivisections, and the tools of the physiologists' trade were those of the chemist and the surgeon. At first microscopes were not to be found: Bichat, for example had no use for them. They began slowly to appear only in the 1830s: 'the new era of microscopic pathological anatomy', wrote Claude Bernard in 1865, 'was originated in Germany by Johannes Müller', with a book published in 1830. Only later, from the 1870s, did bacteriology create a new type of laboratory space, full of microscopes, test tubes, petri dishes, and other types of specialized glassware.

With physiology came another new science, pharmacology (the word dates to 1805). The revolution in chemistry inaugurated by Lavoisier provided the techniques to produce pure samples of the active agents in the plant materials that had been relied on for drug therapy. From Hippocrates on, pharmacists had produced complicated recipes with numerous ingredients. Now, physiologists working with chemists set out to isolate and test one active ingredient at a time. In Germany, morphine was isolated from opium in 1817; in the same year in France emetine was isolated from ipecacuanha root; strychnine was isolated from upas in 1818; quinine from cinchona in 1820; caffeine from coffee in 1821. In 1821 François Magendie published a *Formulaire pour la preparation et l'emploi de plusieurs nouveaux medicamens*. It was 84 pages long. In 1834 the 8th edition appeared; it was 438 pages long. Some of these drugs were certainly useful; but few, perhaps none of them, cured diseases.

Thus by the 1860s medicine appeared to have been transformed: a new relationship between the doctor and the patient's body; a new preoccupation with linking diagnosis and autopsy; new sciences of physiology and pharmacology; and three new locations, first the purpose-built hospital, and then the physiological and the pharmacological laboratories. I wouldn't want to question that there is something profoundly modern about all this, and it certainly was out of this world that modern medicine emerged, but it is essential to stress that the medical revolution represented by the birth of the clinic and of the physiological laboratory was not a success but a failure. The mortality amongst patients did not decrease, instead it increased. New therapies were tried, but they failed. The old complicated pharmacopoeia was abandoned in favour of new, chemically pure drugs which could from the 1850s be injected by hypodermic syringe straight into the bloodstream. Morphine was extracted from opium, quinine was extracted from cinchona, but people went on dying, more or less as before. You could only think that this was the foundation of modern medicine if you thought that modern medicine was about certain institutions (hospitals, laboratories), or certain ways of inspecting patients (stethoscopes, thermometers), or certain ways of interpreting the human body as a prospective cadaver for autopsy (lesions rather than diseases, tissues rather than organs). But if you think that the key feature of modern medicine is effective therapy and the capacity to postpone death, then these institutions, these instruments, this way of thinking about disease are beside the point, because none of them led to effective therapy. The alternative view is that modern medicine began long after the birth of the clinic, and that it is inseparable from the germ theory of disease and the controlled clinical trial.

Why do historians prefer to focus on the birth of the clinic rather than the germ theory of disease or the clinical trial? Part of the answer is that many of them don't actually believe that science progresses. For a relativist, the story of the birth of medical science in the first half of the nineteenth century is a profoundly reassuring one, because the unintended and adverse consequences of so-called progress are far more striking than the intended consequences; doctors, trying hard to save lives, went around killing people. But the story of the birth of the clinic is also attractive to historians because it ties the history of medicine firmly to other sorts of history: the purpose-built hospital can be compared with the prisons and schools being built at the same time (the subject of Foucault's *Discipline and Punish*); the new technically skilled medical professional can be compared with his fellow professionals in law, in the universities, in engineering; experimental physiology is merely one of the new experimental sciences. The problem with the alternative emphasis on the germ theory of disease is not just that it creates a radical discontinuity between the new medicine and the old; it is also that it is much harder to situate this revolution in time and space.

In the story of the birth of the clinic everything can be brought back to the hospital, and the hospital can be given a history. To ask why doctors didn't do better makes little sense. They did what they could in a world that was not of their making. But the story of germ theory is very different. It makes perfect sense to ask why doctors for centuries imagined that their therapies worked when they didn't; why there was a delay of more than two hundred years between the first experiments designed to disprove spontaneous generation and the final triumph of the alternative, the theory that living creatures always come from other living creatures; why there was a delay of two hundred years between the discovery of germs and the triumph of the germ theory of disease; why there was a delay of thirty years between the germ theory of putrefaction and the development of antisepsis; why there was a delay of sixty years between antisepsis and drug therapy. Any history of medicine which focuses on what works immediately brings to the fore these uncomfortable questions about delay, resistance, hostility, and (if we use the word metaphorically) malpractice.

10

THE LABORATORY

Experiments on animals have, we have seen, been central to the development of modern medicine, but some have always found them repugnant, and many have refused to engage in them. The more I have thought about this subject the less sympathetic I have become to all animal experiments conducted before 1877, when Pasteur began work on anthrax. Samuel Johnson said in 1758:

> Among the inferior professors of medical knowledge is a race of wretches, whose lives are only varied by varieties of cruelty . . . What is alleged in defence of these hateful practises everyone knows, but the truth is that by knives, fire, and poison knowledge is not always sought and is very seldom attained. The experiments that have been tried are tried again . . . I know not that by living dissections any discovery has been made by which a single malady is more easily cured. And if knowledge of physiology has been somewhat increased, he surely buys knowledge dear, who learns the use of the lacteals at the expense of his humanity. It is time that universal resentment should arise against these horrid operations . . .

But animal experimentation was absolutely central to the new science of physiology as it developed in the nineteenth century. According to Claude Bernard, the man generally acknowledged as the greatest of all the nineteenth-century physiologists, without vivisection 'neither physiology nor scientific medicine is possible'. Moreover, Bernard was quite explicit in his determination to pay no attention to the pain his animals suffered:

> A physiologist is not a man of fashion, he is a man of science, absorbed by the scientific idea which he pursues: he no longer hears the cry of animals, he no longer sees the blood that flows, he sees only his idea and perceives only organisms concealing problems which he intends to

solve. Similarly, no surgeon is stopped by the most moving cries and sobs, because he sees only his idea and the purpose of his operation. Similarly again, no anatomist feels himself in a horrible slaughter house; under the influence of a scientific idea, he delightedly follows a nervous filament through stinking livid flesh, which to any other man would be an object of disgust and horror.

Bernard was quite right: surgery and anatomy require the overcoming of normal human responses and the substitution of a professional detachment. But Bernard's argument was also a form of special pleading. By the time he wrote this, in 1865, anaesthetics were commonplace. Surgeons no longer had to brace themselves against cries and sobs. As for Bernard he was genuinely indifferent to the sufferings of his animals. One of his research programmes was directed at understanding how curare worked as a poison. Having discovered that it paralysed but did not anaesthetize, Bernard frequently used it to immobilize animals in his experiments, knowing full well that it provided no pain relief. He also understood perfectly that some people found these experiments unbearable to contemplate. His wife left him in 1870, citing his cruelty to animals as a major reason for the break-up of the marriage.

Bernard's famous book *An Introduction to the Study of Experimental Medicine*, from which I have been quoting, was directed at two distinct groups opposed to the new physiology. On the one hand there were the exponents of the statistical method of Louis, who thought that medicine would progress, not by experimenting on animals, but by studying what actually happened to patients. Bernard could scarcely conceal his impatience with such people: 'A great surgeon performs operations for stone by a single method; later he makes a statistical summary of deaths and recoveries, and he concludes from these statistics that the mortality law for this operation is two out of five. Well, I say that this ratio means literally nothing . . .' But Bernard had misrepresented the statistical method: any surgeon announcing a mortality rate of 40 per cent was inviting others to compare their method with his; if their results were worse, they should adopt his method, and if better, he should adopt theirs. Bernard's other imaginary interlocutor was an antivivisectionist. To this person he both presented the arguments for vivisection, and insisted that it was a waste of time doing so, for 'we shall deem all discussion of vivisection futile or absurd'. It is hard not to think that Bernard is here addressing his wife.

Johnson made three charges against vivisection: that it was cruel, that experiments were repeated unnecessarily, and that little of value was learnt from them. For most of the nineteenth century, these remained for many British men and, more frequently, women the key charges against vivisection: I say British, because opposition to vivisection was far stronger in Britain than anywhere else in the world. Even some British vivisectionists were acutely aware of the pain they inflicted on animals in their work. In 1809 Sir Charles Bell conducted pioneering experiments on rabbits to try to establish the function of different nerves in the body—some, it seemed, were primarily employed to convey sensation, others to control movement. The easiest sensation to generate, of course, was pain, but Bell was reluctant to work on conscious rabbits, and stunned his creatures first. 'I cannot perfectly convince myself', he said, 'that I am authorized in nature or religion to do these cruelties—for what?—for anything else than a little egotism or self-aggrandizement; and yet, what are my experiments in comparison with those which are daily done? And done daily for nothing.' As a direct result of this squeamishness he reached the wrong conclusions.

In 1822, the leading French physiologist of the day, François Magendie, repeated Bell's experiments with fully conscious rabbits. He showed that 'the posterior (dorsal) roots of the nerves proceeding from the spinal cord are primarily associated with sensation, whereas the anterior (ventral) roots of the same nerves are primarily associated with motion'. This has been described as the most important single discovery of Magendie's career. It could have been Bell's, but Bell had refused to do the equivalent of learning the use of the lacteals at the expense of his humanity.

At this point, I fear we need to think about actual operations. Sometimes they were straightforwardly elegant, and were not necessarily associated with a great deal of pain. Bernard, who had been Magendie's assistant, developed Magendie's work on the functions of the nerves. One of his studies was of a major nerve in the face, the facial nerve: 'In the first experiment', John Lesch tells us,

> Bernard anaesthetized and immobilized an adult dog with a strong dose of opium extract. He introduced a small hook with a double cutting edge into the skull on the left side via the orifice of the mastoid vein situated above and within the mastoid apophysis. As soon as the instrument had penetrated, Bernard directed it obliquely down and inside, following the posterior face of the petrosal bone. As soon as contractions were visible on the left side of the face, he knew the instrument had reached the facial nerve. Turning the hook upward, and without leaving the petrosal bone, he carefully withdrew the instrument, thereby pulling at and sectioning the nerve. The completion of this operation was signalled by the immediate and complete paralysis of the left side of the face. Within six days the wound had healed and the effects of the opium had dissipated. Bernard was able to confirm that, apart from the facial paralysis, there was a considerable diminution of the gustatory faculty in the left anterior half of the tongue, without any corresponding alteration of movement or of the tactile sense in the same region. When the animal was sacrificed after thirty-three days, autopsy confirmed that the seventh pair, and only the seventh pair, of cranial nerves had been sectioned. He obtained the same results in experiments on two other dogs.

Bernard's study of dogs helped make sense of some cases of facial paralysis in humans: it proved possible to find damage to the facial nerve in an autopsy of a patient whose symptoms were similar to those of the vivisected dogs.

But some operations involved slashing and gashing that caused horrible damage to the dog. Thus Magendie's work on the nerves of the spinal column was conducted on small young dogs. 'He was able to lay bare the membranes of the posterior half of the spinal cord with a single stroke of a very sharp scalpel.' But the shock and blood loss associated with operations such as this were so great that others had difficulty repeating his findings: it turned out that one had to allow the dogs time to recover before manipulating their nerves if one wanted to find what passed for 'normal' physiological responses.

And there is something grotesque about some of the experiments conducted by the French physiologists. Magendie did a good deal of work on the operation of poisons such as strychnine and prussic acid —Bernard was to extend this into studies of curare and carbon monoxide. One question was how poisons such as strychnine, which appeared to work directly on the central nervous system, were absorbed into the body. Was it via the veins, the lacteals, or the nerves? The great eighteenth-century Scottish surgeon John Hunter had done experiments on absorption where he had cut out a small section of a dog's small intestine, leaving it still connected to the blood system and the lacteals, in order to study whether milk was absorbed into the veins or lacteals—he thought he could show that absorption was into the lacteals. Magendie would later seek to disprove this experiment, and show that absorption was into the veins: I'm told by a physiologist that both were right, for the milk's fat would have been absorbed into the lacteals, and the protein and carbohydrates into the veins.

Magendie developed Hunter's experiment: he stripped from the portion of intestine all the vessels until only a single artery and vein were left—strychnine was absorbed into the blood, evidently through the veins in the wall of the gut. He then took this experiment a step further. He severed a dog's leg, leaving it connected to the body by only a single artery and vein. And then he severed these, placing a hollow quill between the two ends—thus the dog and his leg were now connected through an entirely artificial connection, so that no one could argue that there were hidden lacteals that had not been severed. If strychnine was injected into the paw of the severed leg, the dog was poisoned. Conceptually, this experiment was merely a logical development of Hunter's and Magendie's own previous experiments, and yet it seems to me absolutely grotesque, while the other experiments seem merely gruesome. The outcome is the same in both cases: the dog is dead ('sacrificed' is the term of art employed by vivisectionists). It is, I think, the heightened artificiality involved in the severed leg experiment that makes it both perverse and perverted.

In 1824 Magendie visited London where he gave public lectures combined with vivisections. There was what the London Medical Gazette called 'a violent clamour', one with which even a medical journal could sympathize: its word for Magendie's experiments was 'appalling'. In 1837 James Macaulay, an antivivisectionist doctor, attended Magendie's Paris lectures with some friends: 'The whole scene was revolting, not the cruelty only, but the "tiger–monkey" spirit visible in the demoralized students. We left in disgust, and felt thankful such scenes would not be tolerated in England by public opinion.'

The issue of vivisection eventually came to a head in Britain with the publication in 1873 of a book edited by John Burdon Sanderson and entitled *Handbook for the Physiological Laboratory*. This described classic physiological experiments, and was illustrated by numerous photographs. It was clearly intended to bring about a more widespread practice of French-style physiological experimentation in Britain. The book provided immediate evidence in support of the claim that vivisectionists constantly repeated experiments, for it was after all a handbook telling you how to perform experiments that had been performed many times before. Worse, it contained no reference to anaesthesia. Burdon Sanderson later claimed that this was merely an oversight, and the use of anaesthetics was so routine that there had been no need to mention it, but this defence was disingenuous. We now know that Burdon Sanderson and another Englishman, Rutherford, had both performed vivisections using curare and without painkillers.

The furore provoked by the *Handbook* was redoubled when a French physiologist, Eugene Magnan, gave a lecture to the annual meeting of the British Medical Association in August 1874. Magnan had promised to induce the symptoms of epilepsy in dogs by injecting them with absinthe. There were scenes of disorder, and magistrates were called. In February 1875, George Hoggan, who had spent four months working in Bernard's laboratory in Paris, wrote a letter to the *Morning Post* describing the horrors of what he had seen. The result was the establishment of a Royal Commission in 1875. This heard much remarkable testimony. Sir Henry Acland, Regius Professor of Medicine at Oxford and President of the General Medical Council, for example, testified as to the dangers associated with the unprincipled pursuit of knowledge for its own sake. But the star witness turned out to be Emanuel Klein, a German who was working in Britain and was one of the contributors to Burdon Sanderson's handbook. Klein testified that when vivisecting cats and dogs he never bothered with anaesthetics in order to relieve pain; he only employed them when there was risk that he might be bitten or scratched by the suffering animals. After Klein's testimony legislation became inevitable, though what Klein had said was little different from what Bernard had said in his *Introduction*.

The outcome, after much negotiation, was the Cruelty to Animals Act of 1876, the first legislation anywhere in the world to restrict vivisection. The Act provided that anyone experimenting upon living vertebrate animals must have a licence from the Home Secretary; in order to apply for such a licence they must have the support of a president of a major scientific or medical society and of a professor of medicine. The experiments must be performed at a registered location and be open to inspection, and must have as their purpose the acquisition of new knowledge. They must be performed under anaesthesia, and the animal experimented upon must not be revived afterwards. Special licences had to be sought by anyone who intended to experiment without anaesthesia, to repeat experiments that had already been performed, or to use vivisection to illustrate a lecture. Cats, dogs, horses, and donkeys were singled out for particular protection.

In its detail the Act was a commentary on the charges laid against the *Handbook* and the French physiologists. Curare was explicitly ruled not to be an anaesthetic. Obstacles were placed in the way of the repetition of experiments. Many French physiologists had conducted experiments at the Parisian veterinary school of Alfort. There horses that had been condemned to be put down were handed over to students so that they could practise their operative skills upon them, and in Bernard's laboratory animals that still had life in them when the experiments were finished were presented to the students so that they could practise on them. The Act specifically forbade such vivisection to develop manual dexterity. The use of animals in public lectures had caused particular offence in England, and again particular restrictions were placed upon this by the Act.

The Act was an initial success for a strong antivivisection movement which had developed in Britain, and which continued to campaign (indeed continues to campaign) for the complete abolition of vivisection. It was clear from the beginning that the Act would mean whatever the Home Secretary decided it should mean. At first, the Home Secretary acted independently, rejecting a significant number of applications that had the support of the scientific establishment. But in 1881 the International Medical Congress met in London and this meeting was used by the physiologists to mount a campaign against the restrictions being placed upon their work. The timing was perfect. Koch, the discoverer of the life cycle of the anthrax bacillus, was there. So was his rival and enemy Pasteur, who had just demonstrated at Pouilly-Le-Fort the success of his anthrax vaccine: on 31 May fifty sheep, of whom half had previously been vaccinated, were injected with anthrax; on 2 June a large audience (including the correspondent of the London *Times*) could see that all the sheep that had not been vaccinated were either dead or dying, while all but one of the sheep that had been vaccinated were in good health. For the first time, it looked as though experiments on animals might soon open the way to the conquest of human diseases.

In 1882, British physiologists formed the Association for the Advancement of Medicine by Research. At first this was probably envisaged as a campaigning organization to counter the various antivivisectionist societies. But it quickly became something quite different: the Home Secretary agreed that in future the AAMR would inspect all applications for licences to experiment on animals, and that none would be approved without their support; the tacit implication was naturally that applications they supported would be approved. This agreement was reached in private and never publicized. From 1882 the physiologists were in effect allowed to regulate themselves. The Act may have provided some restrictions on their activities and may have required the exercise of a certain caution on their part; but at the same time they were now in a decisive position to control the interpretation of the Act.

What one thinks of this depends in part on whether you think the end justifies the means. In Britain, antivivisectionists and antivaccinationists continued to campaign vigorously against Pasteur's work until the end of the nineteenth century and beyond. But this time the animal experimenters really could point to advances that benefited human beings. And there can be no doubt that the new bacteriology (unlike Jenner's discovery of the smallpox vaccine, which had not involved the death of any animals) was entirely dependent on animal experimentation. Pasteur's work on rabies involved not only infecting dogs with rabies; it also involved infecting rabbits, guinea pigs, and monkeys, in the first two cases to develop virulent strains of rabies, and in the third case to develop an attenuated strain. Dogs that had been rendered immune to rabies were routinely, as Pasteur put it, 'sacrificed' (by injections of strychnine) simply because his laboratory was short of cages and space had to be made for new experimental subjects.

Pasteur's work on rabies provided the model for a younger generation of researchers. In 1894, for example, Yersin published his researches on bubonic plague in Hong Kong. Carrying his 'laboratory' in a small suitcase, working in a tent, in a few weeks he had established that the plague was a disease of rats as well as humans; he had isolated and cultivated the bacillus; he had infected mice, rats, and guinea pigs in the laboratory; and he had learnt how to produce strains of greater and lesser virulence by passing the disease from animal to animal and species to species. Yersin was soon on the track of a vaccine against bubonic plague, a plague that had killed something like 30 per cent of the population of Europe when it had first arrived on the continent in 1348. Triumphs of this sort were impossible without animal experimentation.

Exactly the same argument applies to the first discoveries of effective chemotherapy. Ehrlich's discovery of salvarsan in 1910—the first 'magic bullet' chemical therapy, effective against syphilis—was the result of injecting hundreds of substances into thousands and thousands of infected animals. Salvarsan was the 606th substance on which Ehrlich had carried out animal trials. So too prontosil, the first drug effective against a truly dreadful killer, puerperal fever, which killed women soon after childbirth, was discovered in the Bayer laboratories in 1935 as the result of extensive animal testing. As it happens prontosil was lethal to puerperal fever in the body, but totally ineffective in the test tube, and so could only have been discovered by animal testing—it was later established that prontosil only works because it is broken down in the body into other substances.

English scientists, visiting the Bayer laboratories, were horrified by the numbers of animals killed, and it is significant that early work in England on penicillin involved animal testing on a much smaller scale—the key experiments in Oxford in 1940 involved first eight and then ten mice. In this case the experiments were crucial not in order to show that penicillin was effective against bacteria (that could be shown in the test tube), but to show that it could survive long enough in the body to destroy an infection. Since the production of penicillin was complex and difficult, this knowledge was essential before deciding to scale up production in order to produce sufficient quantities to treat human beings (who are 3,000 times larger than mice).

In defence of the animal experimentalists, one may also say that they were prepared when necessary to experiment upon themselves. The pioneers of anaesthetics had inhaled all sorts of gases to test their effects, and now the bacteriologists followed in their footsteps. When Koch claimed to have identified the cholera vibrio (the name refers to its comma like shape) in 1884 Max von Pettenkofer swallowed a flask full of them—with the intention, it must be said, of proving Koch wrong. (Since he survived, and suffered only from diarrhoea not cholera, he succeeded in casting doubt on Koch's claim.) In 1897 Almroth Wright injected himself and many members of his staff with dead typhoid bacilli to see if they would develop antibodies, which they did. And a volunteer was injected with live bacilli to see if the theoretical immunity worked in practice. In 1928 Alexander Fleming's assistant Stuart Craddock ate penicillin mould to confirm it was not toxic.

It ought to be impossible to discuss vivisection without pausing to ask if it is justified. Can one draw a line, a line which separates the experiments of Bichat, Magendie, and Bernard, who displayed the most callous indifference to animal suffering, from those of Bell, who conscientiously sought to minimize pain, or those of Pasteur and Yersin, of Ehrlich and Domagk (the discoverer of prontosil) which really did save human lives? I'd like to think one can, but who can be trusted, without the benefit of hindsight, to make such distinctions?

JOHN SNOW AND CHOLERA

John Snow's *On the Mode of Communication of Cholera* was published as 'a slender pamphlet' in August 1849, during a major cholera epidemic. It was republished, 'with much new matter', early in 1855, now four times its original length. The pamphlet of 1849 outlined a hypothesis; the book of 1855 demonstrated that hypothesis to be true. Reading it now, it is a breathtaking, an astonishing performance. Yet Snow's arguments were rejected by the leaders of the medical profession, and when, a decade or so later, they came to be generally adopted, they were accepted for the wrong reasons. The response to Snow was a test of his contemporaries, a test they failed.

Snow was the first doctor in the long history of medicine to understand his enemy. He worked out how to prevent cholera, but he did not discover a cure for it. He gave an accurate account of the causal agent, but he never saw it through a microscope. (The first to do so was Filippo Pacini in 1854, though his discovery was largely ignored at the time, and Snow never heard of it.) Snow conducted no experiments, and therefore it is not at first apparent that he was a virtuoso exponent of the experimental method and that the streets of London were his laboratory.

Cholera was a disease unknown to Western Europeans until the late eighteenth century. It began to appear outside Asia, its likely continent of origin, in 1817, and first reached England in 1831, when it killed around 23,000 people. A second outbreak in 1849 killed 53,000. A third, in 1853–4, killed 23,000. A fourth and last, in 1866, killed 14,000. Similar outbreaks occurred across Europe until the end of the nineteenth century. Snow's account of the cause of cholera originated during the second English epidemic and was tested during the third; the adoption of arguments similar to his limited the impact of the fourth epidemic and prevented future epidemics—there were only 135 deaths in England in 1893, when cholera was ravaging much of Europe.

The conventional account of cholera in the 1840s and 1850s held that it was spread as a poison through the air. Like all epidemic diseases, cholera was held to be caused by a miasma, by bad air. (*Malaria* means 'bad air'. Malaria was only shown to be caused by a parasite transmitted by mosquitoes in 1897, so that it remained a disease of bad air long after other diseases, such as cholera, had been shown to be caused by germs.) The ultimate source of bad air was rotting organic matter, and the best way of preventing it therefore was to eliminate the sources of foul odours by improving sewers and drains. Nineteenth-century English reformers such as Edwin Chadwick thus recommended exactly the same improvements that had been urged by their sixteenth-century Italian predecessors. The key difference was that where Renaissance doctors believed that epidemics could under certain circumstances be transmitted directly from one person to another, and so advocated the quarantining of those infected, their nineteenth-century successors held that quarantine measures were pointless, and so allowed the free movement of people and goods even during epidemics: as Snow himself remarked, there were 'great pecuniary interests' that would have been damaged by any recourse to the precautions that had been adopted against the plague.

Snow's starting hypothesis was very different from those of his contemporaries. Because he was a pioneer in the use of anaesthetics (in 1853 he was chosen to administer chloroform to Queen Victoria during the delivery of Prince Leopold), Snow had a great deal of experience in what happened to people and animals when a poison entered the bloodstream as a result of inhalation. (He frequently tried out possible new anaesthetics, first on animals, and then, if the results were promising, on himself.) This experience provided no analogues to cholera. Moreover poisonous gases affected everyone exposed to them, while cholera struck some and passed others by. And poisonous gases obeyed the law of the diffusion of gases:

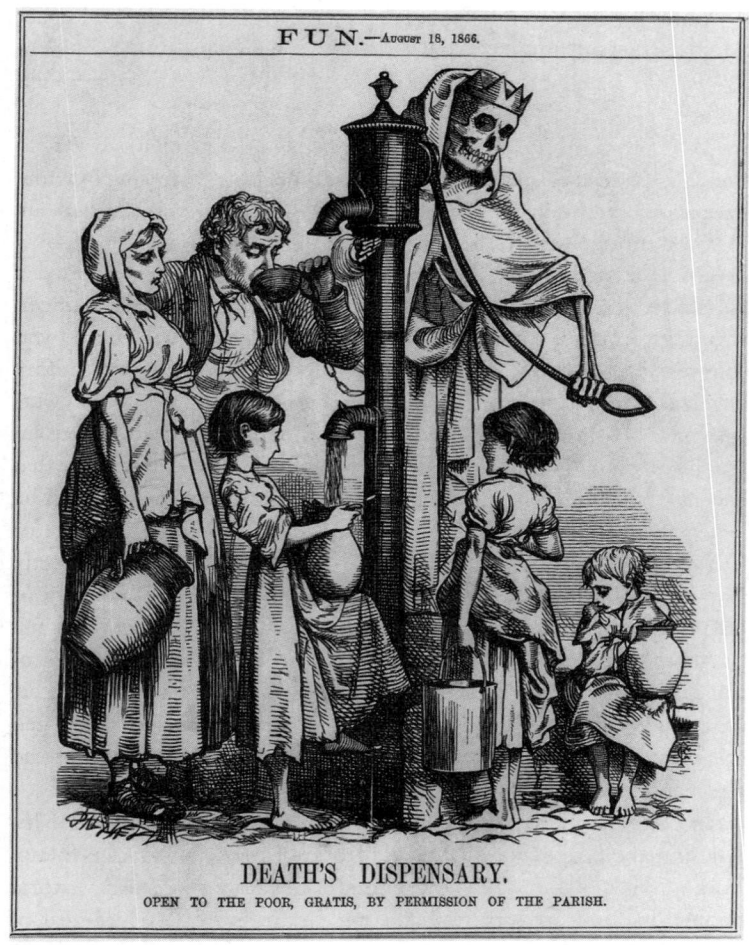

FUN.—August 18, 1866.

DEATH'S DISPENSARY.

OPEN TO THE POOR, GRATIS, BY PERMISSION OF THE PARISH.

27. This drawing by George John Pinwell, entitled *Death's Dispensary*, published in an English magazine during the cholera epidemic of 1866, marks the belated triumph of John Snow's account of the mode of transmission of cholera.

As the gases given off by putrefying substances become diffused in the air, the quantity in a given space is inversely as the square of the distance from their source. Thus a man working with his face one yard from offensive substances would breathe ten thousand times as much of the gas given off as a person living a hundred yards from the spot.

Yet miasmatic theories claimed to be compatible with the fact that people at a considerable distance from the source of a smell often fell ill when those closer to the source were unaffected.

Cholera attacks the gut, causing violent diarrhoea, so Snow concluded it most likely had its origin in something ingested, and this ingested substance probably came more or less directly from cholera sufferers (as smallpox came from smallpox sufferers). Snow was a vegetarian and a teetotaller, and this prepared him for his line of thinking. He himself drank distilled water because he was well aware that one could often find in tap water material that had passed through the human gut. Tap water was not, strictly speaking, vegetarian, since it commonly contained microscopic amounts of half-digested meat. At the age of 17 Snow had read John Frank Newton's *The Return to Nature: A Defence of the Vegetable Regime* (1811), in which the water drunk by Londoners was shown to be full of 'septic matter'. As an anaesthetist, Snow could make no sense of the miasmatic theory's account of how poisonous gases operate; as an admirer of Frank Newton, Snow was predisposed to think that the water people drank made them ill, but he did not develop his alternative theory until the last months of 1848.

In the first edition of *The Mode of Communication of Cholera*, Snow recounts the case of John Barnes, a labourer in Moor Monkton near York, a village untouched by cholera. Barnes's sister had died of cholera in Leeds; two weeks later her clothes were bundled up and sent to Moor Monkton by the carrier. 'The clothes had not been washed; Barnes had opened the box in the evening; on the next day he had fallen sick of the disease.' From John Barnes, the communication of the disease could be traced through twenty individuals (with only one unexplained link), and thirteen deaths. Clearly the disease had travelled in the box of clothes.

Snow had to hand other accounts of the propagation of cholera from person to person. These cases were not compatible with the modification of the miasmatic theory that some advocated, that cholera, originally caused by rotting matter, was also caused by 'effluvia given off from the patient into the surrounding air, and inhaled by others into the lungs'. Snow's alternative hypothesis was that cholera was spread through excreta. The first mode of transmission he identified was from hand to mouth: John Barnes had touched his sister's soiled clothes, had failed to wash his hands, and had conveyed the source of the disease to his own gut. By similar means, his sickness had been conveyed to those who visited him and cared for him. It was easy to show that the disease had an incubation period of twenty-four to forty-eight hours. From the beginning, Snow's argument implied that cholera was an 'animalcule'—although he insisted that all his argument required was that it should be an 'organized particle', one 'capable of multiplying in the human body'. Snow was exploring a germ theory of cholera at a time when germ theories were generally rejected in favour of chemical theories which attributed diseases to poisons (or, to use the Latin term, viruses). He did not want to dismiss out of hand the possibility of some sort of chemical account of the cholera poison, comparable to contemporary accounts of fermentation, which maintained that it was an inorganic process, but his whole argument implied a germ theory, and by 1853 he had committed himself to the view that diseases are caused by living agents.

Snow identified a second mode of transmission, which did not require direct contact with the patient or their personal effects. He looked closely at two identical alleys of houses in Horsleydown, near London, that stood next to each other. Cholera had struck one alleyway, called Surrey Buildings, killing eleven people, and had almost entirely spared the other, killing only one. In the alleyway where the infection had spread overflow from the drains ran back into the well from which the inhabitants drew their water. The soiled clothes of the sick had been washed in water that their neighbours had then drunk. Cholera had spread through the pollution of the water supply.

In another case, a London suburban development called Albion Terrace, Snow had identified a row of seventeen houses where a severe rainstorm had caused the cesspools to overflow into the water supply. Here twenty-four people had died. In a neighbouring house, supplied with the same water, a gentleman who had always refused to drink the water was untouched. In 1849, Snow had five other examples of disease hotspots that could only be explained by the hypothesis that cholera was entering the drinking water. One was of a landlord who had dismissed his tenants' complaints that their water stank. Cholera was frequent amongst the tenants, but not in the distant village where the landlord lived. One Wednesday he drank a glass of his tenants' water to show there was nothing wrong with it; he died the following Saturday.

The official account of the deaths at Albion Terrace blamed an open sewer 400 feet away, which caused an unpleasant smell when the wind was in the wrong direction, together with a disagreeable smell from the sinks in the houses and some smelly rubbish in the basement of one of the houses. In other words the orthodox explanation was that the disease was airborne, and that it was caused (as all epidemic diseases had been believed to have been caused for centuries) by the smell of putrefaction. The solution was improved hygiene. Snow pointed out that most of London was exposed to exactly the same sorts of smells that were to be found at Albion Terrace, but on other such streets nobody at all had died.

Snow had rejected the conventional view that cholera was transmitted through the air and was primarily caused by putrefaction. Instead he argued that it was transmitted through the water supply and by direct contact, and was carried in the faeces of cholera sufferers. He was thinking in terms of a germ theory of the disease. The great advantage of this was that he could explain why cholera seemed to strike in a random fashion. If it was dissolved in the air (as Haygarth thought the poison that caused smallpox was) or in the water, then it should affect everyone, or everyone who used that water, more or less identically. But if it was some sort of living creature, however small, then one glass of water might contain the infection, while another, equally impure in other respects (Snow found bits of skin and hair in the piped water supply), might not. 'The eggs of the tape-worm must undoubtedly pass down the sewers into the Thames, but it by no means follows that everybody who drinks a glass of the water should swallow one of the eggs.' The germ theory was thus crucial to explaining the erratic or seemingly random incidence of the disease.

Snow's appeal to tape-worms seems obvious and straightforward to us, but the question of whether parasitic worms were spontaneously generated was still being debated in the 1840s. A key text arguing against spontaneous generation was J. J. S. Steenstrup's *On the Alternation of Generations* (1845), which gave an account of the life cycle of the liver fluke. Snow's contemporaries had thus only just caught up with Leeuwenhoek and Swammerdam, who had been convinced that the microscope opened the way to a refutation of spontaneous generation. It is also significant that infection by tape-worms had been used as an analogy for germ infection by Jacob Henle in *Pathologische Untersuchungen* (1840), the most important defence of germ theory before Pasteur, precisely in order to explain the apparently random incidence of diseases. Snow never refers to Henle directly, but he may well have read him.

Snow saw that it was possible to test his hypothesis that cholera was transmitted through drinking water on a larger scale. In some parts of London water was supplied from the Thames, into which most sewers emptied. The Thames is a tidal river, so sewage would have been carried up the river as well as down; even where water was drawn from a source above the sewage outfall it would have been polluted with sewage so long as it was not drawn from a point above the highest reach of the tide. Some companies filtered the water they drew from the Thames or passed it through settling pools, some did not. Yet other companies drew their water from uncontaminated springs. It was thus a simple matter to compare the incidence of cholera in particular districts with the supply of drinking water in those districts. In Southwark, in 1832, water was taken straight from the Thames without filter or settling reservoir. The death rate was 110 per 10,000. In equally poor Shoreditch, water came mainly from the New River and the River Lea. The death rate was 10 per 10,000. Exactly comparable results applied in 1849.

The careful case studies Snow produced of transmission from person to person and from house to house were highly suggestive, as was the comparative work he did on the incidence of cholera amongst the customers of different water companies, but since his conclusions were directly opposed to the long tradition of Hippocratic medicine, with its single-minded emphasis on miasma or bad air, it is hardly surprising that his contemporaries found them unconvincing. As far as Snow was concerned the return of cholera in 1853 was to provide a perfect opportunity to test his arguments. Snow's most important study during the epidemic of 1853–4 was a comparative analysis of the incidence of cholera amongst the customers of different water companies. Since one of the companies had changed its source of water, he could show that the general pattern was comparable to those for 1832 and 1849, with the major change that his hypothesis would have predicted, that an improvement in the purity of water had led directly to a decline in the incidence of cholera—and he could show that similar changes had taken place in Glasgow and Hull when water companies altered their sources of supply.

In general, in London different companies served different areas. But in some areas two companies were in direct competition with each other, with one house drawing water from one company, and its neighbour from another. This, Snow said, was the equivalent of a laboratory experiment to test his theory:

> As there is no difference whatever, either in the houses or the people receiving the supply of the two Water Companies, or in any of the physical conditions with which they are surrounded, it is obvious that no experiment could have been devised which would more thoroughly test the effect of water supply on the progress of cholera than this, which circumstances placed ready made before the observer.

> The experiment, too, was on the grandest scale. No fewer than three hundred thousand people of both sexes, of every age and occupation, and of every rank and station, from gentlefolks down to the very poor, were divided into two groups without their choice, and, in most cases, without their knowledge; one group being supplied with water containing the sewage of London and the other group having water quite free from such impurity.

Snow and an associate set out to visit every house in which there had been a cholera fatality and establish which company supplied its water—Snow cut back on his practice, effectively giving up his income, in order to pursue his enquiries. Between 8 July and 5 August 1854 there were 563 deaths from cholera in London, or 9 deaths per 10,000 houses. In 40,046 houses supplied by the polluted water of the Southwark and Vauxhall Co. there were 286 fatalities, or 71 per 10,000 houses. Amongst the identical houses intermingled amongst them but supplied with the clean water of the Lambeth Co. there were 14 fatalities, or 5 per 10,000. Note that these fourteen fatalities did not present a problem for Snow's argument: it was to be expected that some customers of the Lambeth Co. would visit friends who were customers of the Southwark and Vauxhall Co. and drink their water; would purchase drinks made with Southwark and Vauxhall water in pubs and cafés; and would visit and nurse those who had fallen sick from drinking Southwark and Vauxhall water.

Snow's use of the customers of the two water companies as a randomized trial of his hypothesis resulted in a brilliant vindication of his arguments. (Snow's survey was later repeated and extended with much less striking results. But it is Snow's results that are to be trusted. He published a list running over twenty-five pages of every death and every address in his study; and he pointed out two major difficulties: there was often more than one house with the same street address, so that one had to make careful enquiries to make sure one was at the right address; and people often did not know the name of their water supplier, since that was a matter for their landlord—a problem Snow had circumvented by devising a chemical test to distinguish the water supplies of the two companies.) Snow also showed that an analysis of the occupations of those who died from cholera was highly revealing. Sailors and ballast-heavers were accustomed to drink water direct from the Thames—one in twenty-four of them died of cholera in the epidemic of 1848–9; those who worked in breweries were said never to drink water at all, and indeed none of them died.

Contemporaries often implied that it really did not matter whether Snow was right or not. Both the miasmatists and Snow believed that human faeces helped spread cholera, so one could conclude from both their arguments that improved sanitation was the answer. Snow was impatient with this response, as he held that the activities of those who advocated improved sanitation had had the opposite effect from the one they had intended. In 1854, publishing the preliminary results of his enquiry into the water supply, he wrote:

> The persons who have been more instrumental in causing the increase in cholera are precisely those who have made the greatest efforts to check it, and who have been loudest in blaming the supineness of others. In 1832 there were few water-closets in London. The privies were chiefly emptied by night men, a race who have almost ceased to exist; or a portion of the contents of the cesspool flowed slowly, and after a time, into the sewers. By continued efforts to get rid of what were called the removable causes of disease, the excrement of the community has been washed every year more rapidly into the river from which two-thirds of the inhabitants, till lately, obtained their supply of water. While the faeces lay in the cesspools or sewers, giving off a small quantity of unpleasant gas having no power to produce specific diseases, they were spoken of as dangerous and pestilential nuisances; but when washed into the drinking-water of the community, they figured only in Sanitary Reports as so many grains of organic matter per gallon.

Thus the difference between his own account of the transmission of the disease and that of the miasmatists was fundamental. His priority was clean drinking water; theirs was flush toilets.

Just as Snow had studied both the customers of water companies and particular hotspots in 1849, so now in 1854 he did a detailed study of one particular hotspot, in Broad Street, by Golden Square. There, within a circle with a radius of two hundred and ten yards, five hundred people died of cholera within ten days, between 31 August and 9 September. In the first two days, 197 people died. The next day Snow interrupted his survey of water company customers to study this outbreak. He immediately looked for a possible source of contaminated water, and his attention focused on a pump in Broad Street, by Golden Square, which stood roughly at the centre of the outbreak. He had no direct proof that the water was polluted (it was not until six months later that Henry Whitehead was to show that the first case had been that of a baby girl, and that the water in which her nappies had been washed had gone into a drain which leaked into the well). What he could do was trace the 83 people who had died in the immediate neighbourhood during the previous three days and whose deaths had been registered (of the 197 deaths others had not yet been registered or had occurred in hospitals outside the neighbourhood); of these he could show that 77 had almost certainly drunk water from the pump. Four days after he arrived in the neighbourhood, a week after the beginning of the outbreak, Snow asked the local authority, the parish vestry, to remove the handle from the pump. This they did; the outbreak was already diminishing (for the water was probably no longer polluted), and within twenty-four hours it was effectively over.

In the 2nd edition of *The Mode of Communication of Cholera* Snow published a map of the fatalities and their relationship to the Broad Street pump and to the other pumps in the neighbourhood. In another version of the map he even drew a dotted line which enclosed all the places which were closer to the Broad Street pump than to any other: the line follows a complicated path, allowing for the fact that pedestrians, unlike birds, cannot take the shortest route between two points, but must follow streets and turn corners. (This is now called a Voronoi diagram, and Snow's map is the first such diagram.) Nearly all the deaths fell within the dotted line.

The story of the pump handle and the map that illustrates it have entered the folklore of epidemiology, though the often careless retelling of this story has opened the way to a fundamental misunderstanding of what Snow had accomplished. No map showing Broad Street and its immediate area to be a hotspot, it is said, could prove Snow's account of how cholera was transmitted; for other contemporaries produced similar maps, and they were convinced that such maps showed that the disease was most likely disseminated through the air. They hypothesized some unidentified source of miasma at the centre of the circle within which the deaths fell. Consequently, it is argued, Snow had failed to prove his case, and his opponents had at least as good an argument as he had. But this is to make the elementary mistake of imagining that the map was a full presentation of Snow's material—ignoring not only the other evidence we have so far surveyed, but the fact that Snow had crucial additional evidence relating to the Broad Street epidemic itself.

The workhouse in Poland Street was near the epicentre of the

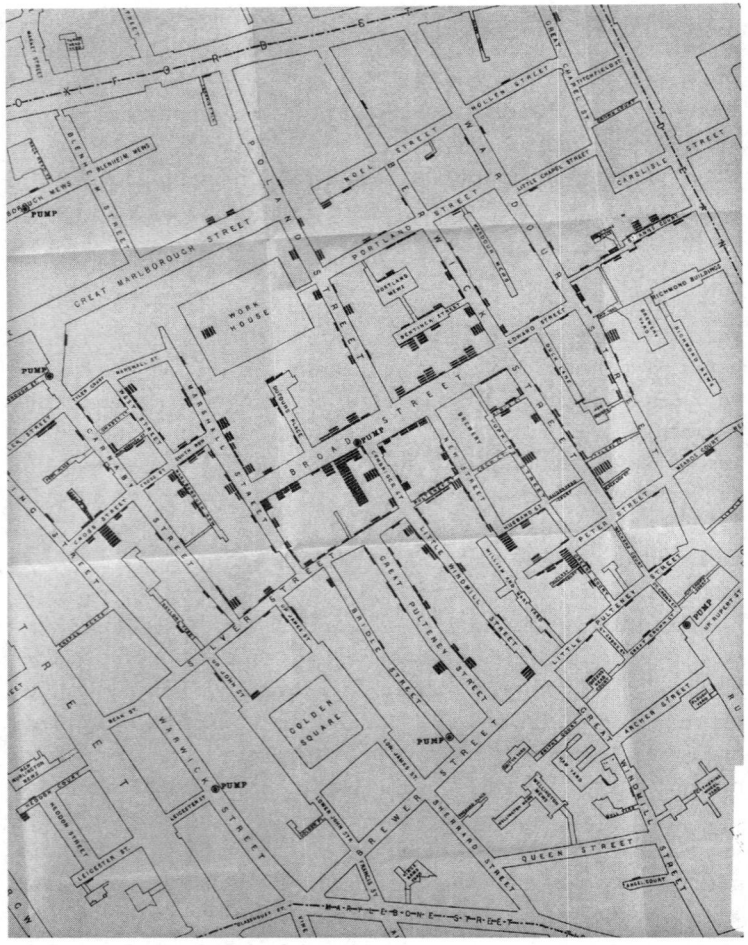

28. The map of the fatalities in the neighbourhood of the Broad Street pump from the second edition of Snow's *The Mode of Communication of Cholera*.

hotspot. It had 535 inmates but only 5 fatalities. The inmates breathed the air of Broad Street, but did not drink water from its pump. On Broad Street itself a brewery employed 70 men; none of them died. All drank beer not water; in any case the brewery had its own well. At a percussion cap factory a few yards away 18 of 200 workers died; they were supplied with water from the pump. Both those who worked in the brewery and those who worked in the percussion cap factory breathed the same air, but they did not drink the same water. One person, who came from Brighton, spent twenty minutes in the house of someone who had died of cholera, drank a glass of brandy diluted with water from the Broad Street pump, and died the next day. A woman who lived in Hampstead, an area untouched by cholera, and who never went to Broad Street, but who was regularly supplied with a bottle of water from the Broad Street pump (she had lived in the area in the past and thought the water particularly delicious) died, as did her niece, who drank from the same bottle—Snow describes this case (which of necessity does not appear on his map) as 'perhaps the most conclusive of all in proving the connexion between the Broad Street pump and the outbreak of cholera'. The point being that the man from Brighton, the widow from Hampstead, together with her niece who was from Islington, did not breathe Broad Street air, but died just the same because they drank Broad Street water. No hypothesis, other than Snow's, could account for their deaths. The map was not a complete representation of Snow's argument; it was merely an illustration of one part of it.

If any epidemiological study could be conclusive, Snow's was—the standard modern objection to epidemiological studies is that they are not randomized, but Snow's study of the area of London where two water companies supplied water in competition with each other amounted to a randomized study. Henry Whitehead, the local clergyman, who set out on a house to house enquiry in order to refute Snow's argument, ended up being converted to it. And yet his conclusions were not accepted. Two enquiries—one instituted by the Metropolitan Commission of Sewers, and the other by the Committee on Scientific Enquiries of the General Board of Health, representing the national government—ruled in favour of airborne contagion.

The Committee on Scientific Enquiries was particularly impressed by a study by William Farr, which showed a very close correlation in London and to some degree elsewhere in England between the death rate from cholera and proximity to sea level—Farr even produced a mathematical formula to show that at half the elevation the mortality doubled, and so forth: thus the mortality was in the inverse ratio of the elevation. This formula would have resulted in the death of each and every person who happened to live exactly at sea level, but Farr pointed out that buildings raise us above the ground, so that the inhabitants of buildings at sea level, he claimed, actually lived (presumably he meant slept) at a height of 13 feet above sea level. He combined such mathematical exactitude with much pure nonsense. 'On the high lands,' he writes, 'men feel the loftiest emotions . . . Man feels his immortality in the hills.' Hence all religions associate their gods with hills, not with swamps. Farr feared that the English were increasingly living in cities close to sea level, which would result in the degeneration of the race and the collapse of the population. The government should force people to build on higher ground.

Snow had already effectively demolished Farr when the Committee on Scientific Enquiries declared its support for him: 'Dr Farr', says Snow,

> was inclined to think that the level of the soil had some direct influence over the prevalence of cholera, but the fact of the most elevated towns in this kingdom, as Wolverhampton, Dowlais, Merthyr Tydvil, and Newcastle-upon-Tyne, having suffered excessively from this disease on several occasions, is opposed to this view, as is also the circumstance of Bethlehem Hospital, the Queen's Prison, Horsemonger Lane Gaol, and several other large buildings, which are supplied with water from deep wells on the premises, having nearly or altogether escaped cholera, though situated on a very low level, and surrounded by the disease . . .

Farr's low-lying towns struck by cholera were, any reader of Snow will recognize, towns that drew water from tidal rivers. Farr was not wrong to think there was some sort of correlation between height above sea level and the incidence of cholera; his mistake lay in assuming that the difference was in the air people breathed not the water they drank.

Of all the objections made to Snow there is only one that presented any difficulty for Snow's argument. If cholera could be spread from hand to mouth, why did doctors (who often conducted autopsies on cholera victims) and undertakers (who handled their bodies) not fall ill as frequently as the relatives of the sick? Snow's answer was that doctors and undertakers took care to wash their hands—for him this constituted evidence that the simplest of precautions could serve to keep cholera at bay.

There were two people whom Snow needed to convince. One was his opponent William Farr, who was superintendent of the statistical department of the General Register Office, and the acknowledged expert on the use of statistics in the study of diseases. As we have seen, in the 1850s he had an alternative theory; by 1866 however he was a convert to Snow's germ theory, and he played a leading role in showing that the 1866 cholera epidemic was water-borne. The other was John Simon, who was Medical Officer of Health to the Privy Council, and the authority on whom the government relied. Simon was happy to accept that water played a role in the dissemination of cholera, but he thought it was only one factor amongst many. He too converted in 1866, claiming that the decisive evidence was not the 'popular' experiment (that is, 'the experiments which accident does for us') 'performed on half a million human beings in South London by the commercial water companies' but the 'scientific' experiment of Karl Thiersch.

Thiersch, working in Germany, took fresh intestinal liquid from cholera victims. He allowed it to decompose by exposure to air. He then fed small quantities to mice. He found that fresh faecal matter was harmless, as was faecal matter that had stood around for a week or so, but faecal matter that was three or four days old was deadly. The mice, Thiersch claimed, had successfully been infected with cholera. Thiersch's work was immediately publicized by Justus von Liebig, the greatest biochemist of the day, who held the view that diseases were caused by poisons. From Simon's point of view the great attraction of this experiment was that it explained why doctors and undertakers, who encountered relatively fresh faecal matter, were not infected. But there are several problems with Simon's conversion as a result of

Thiersch's experiment. The first is that the experiment had been conducted as early as 1854, and indeed had been rejected by Snow in his 2nd edition. Snow was sure the experiment was faulty because he knew the incubation period of the disease was only twenty-four to forty-eight hours—there was no time for the three or four day period of putrefaction posited by Thiersch. The second is that we now know you cannot give mice cholera by feeding them cholera germs. So whatever Thiersch had done, he had not infected his mice with cholera.

Nevertheless, in 1866 Simon had Thiersch's experiments repeated in England and declared them decisive. Why? What had changed was not the evidence regarding the transmission of cholera, which was exactly the same as it had been when Snow published his 2nd edition. What had changed was the acceptability of miasmatic theories of disease. Villemin had shown that tuberculosis could be transmitted from one animal to another. Sanderson had done similar work with cattle plague. Pasteur's work was beginning to be widely discussed— it was known to Farr. The medical profession was on the point of abandoning its commitment to miasmatic theories of epidemics and of adopting the view that each disease had a specific agent, even if it had yet to make a choice between Leibig's view, that the agent was chemical, and Pasteur's, that it was living. Farr and Simon were simply dedicated followers of fashion. This time, for a change, the fashionable view happened to be the right one.

12
PUERPERAL FEVER

Puerperal fever or childbed fever is (we now know) a bacterial infection of the genital tract, often leading to peritonitis and a dreadfully painful death. In the eighteenth and nineteenth centuries some 6 to 9 women in every 1,000 deliveries succumbed to puerperal fever, and just under half that number died. Epidemics sometimes occurred for unknown reasons, especially in maternity hospitals, and then the rate of infection soared and the proportion of those who died reached 80 per cent. In the General Lying-In Hospital, London, between 1835 and 1844 there were on average 63 deaths for every 1,000 deliveries. The most common treatment was, of course, bleeding, but some doctors also recognized that no treatment was of any help. Thus in the early nineteenth century William Hunter said 'Of those attacked by this disease, treat them in any manner you will, at least three out of four will die.' Cause and cure were both equally mysterious.

In 1795 an obscure doctor in Aberdeen, Alexander Gordon, published an account of an epidemic of puerperal fever that had occurred in the town between late 1789 and spring 1792. Gordon had studied in London, which meant that he was confident he was familiar with the literature on puerperal fever, and he had the confidence to decide that it was wrong. In the course of the epidemic he reached three conclusions. First, he realized that the disease was contagious: this involved rejecting the conventional view that epidemics of puerperal fever, like all epidemics, were a result of some noxious quality in the air. Moreover he recognized that it was spread by doctors and midwives from one patient to another: it 'seized such women only as were visited or delivered by a practitioner, or taken care of by a nurse, who had previously attended patients affected by the disease'. As the epidemic developed he became able to predict who would come down with the disease because he had worked out which doctors, midwives, and nurses were carrying it.

He himself, Gordon realized, was one of those spreading the disease. Since the infectious disease that was best understood was smallpox, which is airborne, and since epidemics were always assumed to be airborne, he assumed the infection was in the atmosphere surrounding a person, and clung, as a smell would, to their clothes. Thus the patient's clothes and bedclothes should be either burnt or 'thoroughly purified', and those who had attended the patient 'ought carefully to wash themselves and to get their apparel properly fumigated before it be put on again'. Second, he saw that there was a close relationship between puerperal fever and erysipelas, an infection of the skin, usually of the face. Erysipelas is normally painful but not life-threatening, but it can develop into streptococcal septicaemia, or even into what is now called necrotizing fasciitis (or 'flesheating disease') and was once called gangrenous erysipelas. In the eighteenth and nineteenth centuries erysipelas killed about the same number of people as did puerperal fever. In Aberdeen, the epidemic of puerperal fever was in some manner connected to an epidemic of erysipelas, 'for these two epidemics began in Aberdeen at the same time, and afterwards kept pace together; they both arrived at their acme together, and they both ceased at the same moment'. Finally, he argued that early, copious, and repeated bleeding could be effective as a cure. He could indeed show that as the epidemic went on, and as he turned to more vigorous bleeding, the death rate fell—he was not to know that this is a common feature of epidemics.

When Gordon published his account of the epidemic a storm broke over his head. He had named those (including himself) who had been spreading the disease, and the numbers each had killed, ensuring he had a number of vocal enemies. And his enemies claimed that the cause of the high death rate was not the disease at all: they had never heard of puerperal fever before Gordon's arrival, and took these to be cases of minor infection that had unaccountably turned fatal. No, the cause of the deaths was Gordon's excessive bleeding. Gordon was forced to abandon his practice, and died soon afterwards at the age of 47. His little book however established itself in the medical literature, not because he had argued that puerperal fever was contagious (an argument that made no sense to his contemporaries), nor because he had linked puerperal fever to erysipelas (others were to make this link without acknowledging Gordon, and by 1849 Fleetwood Churchill felt it reasonable to conclude that puerperal fever and erysipelas were 'essentially the same disease'), but because he appeared to have provided decisive evidence on a much debated question: how much to bleed.

In May 1842 a meeting of the College of Physicians of Philadelphia discussed both a recent outbreak of erysipelas and a recent outbreak of puerperal fever. One doctor, Dr Rutter, had had no less than seventy patients with puerperal fever during 1841–2. He ceased practice for several weeks, washed thoroughly, shaved his head and face, changed his clothes and equipment; yet when he resumed the infections resumed until he eventually left Philadelphia. In Boston too there was a discussion of puerperal fever, caused by the case of a doctor who had examined the corpse of someone who had died of puerperal fever, and who had then himself died, along with several of his obstetrical patients. Oliver Wendell Holmes, a young doctor present at the discussion, offered to research the question, and published a paper on the subject in an obscure journal in 1843, reprinting it as a pamphlet under the title *Puerperal Fever as a Private Pestilence* in 1855.

Holmes collected together, with remarkable and scrupulous care, all the evidence that puerperal fever was contagious, vindicating Gordon's argument. He also confirmed Gordon's link between puerperal fever and erysipelas. He carefully avoided theorizing: 'Where facts are numerous, and unquestionable, and unequivocal in their significance, theory must follow them as it best may, keeping time with their step, and not go before them, marching to the sound of its own drum and trumpet.' And he accepted conventional miasmatic explanations. It was, he said, an

undisputed fact, that within the walls of lying-in hospitals there is often generated a miasm, palpable as the chlorine used to destroy it, tenacious so as in some cases almost to defy extirpation, deadly in some institutions as the plague, which has killed women in a private hospital of

London so fast that they were buried two in one coffin to conceal its horrors . . .

And he presented a simple set of recommendations: no doctor with an obstetrical practice should ever conduct an autopsy on a case of puerperal fever. Any physician who had 'three or more closely connected cases of puerperal fever should regard it as prima facie evidence that he is the vehicle of contagion'. To carry on delivering babies in such circumstances was, in moral terms, to commit murder. It was 'professional homicide'.

Holmes's conclusions were naturally unacceptable to many of his contemporaries. Charles Meigs, who held the chair of midwifery and diseases of women at Jefferson College, dismissed his arguments as the 'maunderings of a sophomore'. As far as Meigs was concerned, Dr Rutter's unfortunate experience was one of pure bad luck. This was not the only occasion on which Holmes found himself under attack from his professional colleagues, and it might be tempting to hold them responsible for his decision to give up medical practice and turn to writing poetry and delivering public lectures: except for the fact that Holmes continued to lecture on physiology at Harvard until the normal retirement age. If his relationship with the medical profession was deeply uncomfortable, it was never entirely broken.

Holmes, like Gordon, had no idea how the disease was carried from doctor to patient. All that was apparent was that it was. In 1850 James Simpson suggested a new way of drawing an analogy between puerperal fever and the best understood of the infectious diseases, smallpox. He suggested that:

> patients during labour have been and may be locally inoculated with a *materies morbi* [infectious matter] capable of exciting puerperal fever; that this *materies morbi* is liable to be inoculated into the dilated and abraded lining membrane of the maternal passages during delivery by the fingers of the attendant; that thus in transferring it from one patient to another, the fingers of the attendant act, as it were, like the ivory points formerly used by some of the early vaccinators . . .

Thus puerperal fever was caused by the introduction of diseased matter, from other cases of puerperal fever, or erysipelas, or gangrene, into the abraded lining of the uterus. It was thus spread both in the same way in which smallpox was spread by innoculators, and in the same way that infections were spread during surgery. The title of Simpson's paper was 'Some notes on the analogy between puerperal fever and surgical fever'.

When Simpson's paper appeared in 1850, Ignaz Semmelweis, a young Hungarian appointed an assistant in the lying-in hospital in Vienna, was propounding a rather different account of puerperal fever. Unlike Gordon, Holmes, and Simpson, Semmelweis has become a hero, at least in the eyes of some, the first proponent, it is said, of a modern theory of infection.

Vienna had the largest lying-in hospital in the world, with about 7,000 deliveries a year. The hospital was opened in 1784; in 1833 two admissions wards were established, admitting on alternate days; and from 1839 one of these wards was used for teaching all the male medical students, and the other for teaching all the female midwives. From that point on the mortality rate from puerperal fever (which had previously been identical in the two clinics) was much higher in the first clinic, where the men were taught, than in the second clinic, where the women were taught. Semmelweis, who established these facts, also established there had been a general increase in mortality after 1823. This was the moment when it became routine to teach medical students through the post-mortem dissection of cadavers. Semmelweis could see only one explanation for the increase in mortality after 1823 and the differential mortality between the two wards after 1839: male medical students, who frequently handled cadavers, were bringing the cause of the disease on their hands from the morgue to the wombs of their patients. In particular he saw a striking similarity between the symptoms of puerperal fever and the symptoms exhibited by Professor Kolletschka, a forensic pathologist who died of blood poisoning following an accidental injury while conducting an autopsy. Mothers dying from puerperal fever were dying for the same reason that Kolletschka had died—cadaveric material was entering their bloodstreams. This hypothesis also helped to explain a number of puzzling features of the incidence of puerperal fever. Puerperal fever was rare among mothers who delivered prematurely or who were brought to the hospital immediately after delivery—but these mothers were the only ones who were not subjected to internal examinations by students.

In May 1847 Semmelweis required everyone to wash their hands with chloride of lime (which eliminated the smell of the dissecting room) before beginning to examine living patients. At once, the incidence of puerperal fever fell sharply. Semmelweis had recognized that (since patients were divided randomly between the two wards) the difference in mortality between the two wards must be due to some difference in the treatment of patients on the two wards. The difference evidently had something to do with the difference between male medical and female midwifery students; and the only obvious difference was that the first conducted autopsies and the second did not. This observation had enabled him to eliminate the major cause of puerperal fever in the Vienna lying-in hospital. But six months later there was a new outbreak. Semmelweis traced it to a woman with cancer of the uterus. Students examined her, and then in turn the women in beds next to hers—eleven out of twelve of them then died from puerperal fever. Clearly living patients could produce infectious material similar to that produced by corpses. Semmelweis now believed puerperal fever was an infection of the blood caused by decomposing animal organic matter, and now required disinfectant washings after the examination of patients suffering from conditions other than pregnancy.

In some cases (perhaps in 200 of 10,000 live births), Semmelweis believed decomposition could take place within the woman's uterus, as a result, for example, of the retention of part of the placenta. These women would self-infect, causing a low, largely inescapable, sporadic incidence of puerperal fever and a death rate of under 1 per cent of deliveries. The primary task of doctors was to eliminate external causes of infection, bringing the death rate down to its irreducible minimum.

Semmelweis had produced two accounts of puerperal fever—the cadaveric matter account, and the decomposing animal organic matter account. The two were sufficiently similar to be easily confused with each other, but it was the first, 'the theory of cadaverous infection', which gained most attention and unfortunately was open to fairly straightforward objections, as cases of puerperal fever were often found where neither doctors nor midwives had conducted autopsies. The second account made it difficult to understand why every delivery did not result in puerperal fever, for did not all doctors treat patients with diseases of one sort or another? The result was a fair amount of confusion as to what Semmelweis was claiming, and Semmelweis did not help matters by relying on others to report his achievements: he did not publish anything himself until 1856 (a lecture printed in a Budapest medical journal), and did not publish a sustained account of his work until 1860, thirteen years after he had reduced the death rate in Vienna. Despite the fact that he had a number of prominent supporters in Vienna, he had failed to obtain secure employment there, and had returned to Budapest in 1850. He began work on his great treatise in 1857, but already his behaviour was beginning to seem eccentric, and the treatise itself suggests someone under enormous strain. By 1861 he was denouncing those who had not adopted his views as murderers. In 1865 he attended a meeting to report on a vacant appointment; instead he read out the text of the midwives' oath. A week later, he was taken to Vienna and put in a lunatic asylum. He tried to escape, and was restrained; two weeks later he died. The cause of death was blood poisoning from an infected finger—the finger, according to the death certificate, had been infected during a gynaecological examination. Semmelweis had died of septicaemia, a condition that he would have held to be identical to puerperal fever.

It is not surprising that there has been a good deal of speculation about the cause of Semmelweis's mental breakdown. Some blame Alzheimer's, some syphilis, some manic-depressive psychosis with paranoid features. It seems to me important to bear in mind Semmelweis's obsession with the vast numbers of needless deaths from puerperal fever. This was a subject to which he returned constantly in his lectures: 'often, when speaking to his class, his excitement rose to such a degree as to cause alarm to those around him'.

We need to take seriously the enormous pressure upon people such as Snow, Gordon, Holmes, and Semmelweis. They believed they

TABLE 3. Puerperal fever in the Vienna Lying-In Hospital, 1784–1859

	Births	Deaths	Rate
Before pathological anat-omy (1784–1823)	71,395	897	1.25%
After pathological anatomy (1823–33)	28,429	1,509	5.3%
Two identical wards: ward 1 (1833–41)	23,059	1,505	6.56%
Two identical wards: ward 2 (1833–41)	13,097	731	5.58%
Ward 1, male students, no chlorine washings (1841–7)	20,042	1,989	9.92%
Ward 2, female students, no chlorine washings (1841–7)	17,791	691	3.38%
Ward 1, male students, since chlorine washings (1849–59)	47,938	1,712	3.57%
Ward 2, female students, since chlorine washings (1849–59)	40,770	1,248	3.06%
75 year totals	262,523	10,282	3.91%

knew how to prevent deaths that were occurring around them. Snow reacted to this pressure with great care and restraint. We feel its presence only in occasional carefully formulated asides, as when he says that

It may, indeed, be confidently asserted, that if the Southwark and Vauxhall Water Company had been able to use the same expedition as the Lambeth Company in completing their new works, and obtaining water free from the contents of sewers, the late epidemic of cholera would have been confined in a great measure to persons employed among the shipping and to poor people who get water by pailsfull direct from the Thames or tidal ditches.

He provides a useful table which enables us to see that 4,093 deaths were directly attributable to the Southwark and Vauxhall Co.—and every one of these deaths was also, alas, attributable to John Snow's failure to produce a sufficiently convincing case in 1849 to change government policy.

We see the pressure more obviously at work in Holmes, who refused to reply to Charles Meigs's attacks, saying 'No man makes a quarrel with me over the counterpane that covers a [dying] mother, with her new-born infant at her breast.' Nevertheless, he had made clear that men like Meigs were guilty of murder. In the case of Semmelweis the pressure was obviously more than he could bear. He saw himself as dealing with an obstinate refusal to accept the truth, a determination to cling to 'a theory that condemns to death those who are cared for as required by that theory, and indeed, achieves their deaths by the hands of those who are taught to save them'. He compared the mortality rate amongst his own patients with the mortality rate amongst the patients of a Dr Lumpe: 'Dr Lumpe explains the origin of puerperal fever by epidemic influences and he sends nearly one patient to the morgue each day. I explain the origin of puerperal fever by infection with decaying matter and in 1848 I sent only forty-five patients to the morgue.' He tells the story of Professor Michaelis from Kiel, who had written to him 'Last summer my cousin died of puerperal fever. I had examined her after delivery at a time when I had autopsied patients who had died of puerperal fever. From that time I was convinced of communicability.' Unable to bear the responsibility of having killed his cousin, 'he sank into a deep melancholy, and threw himself under a train speeding into Hamburg. I have related', says Semmelweis, 'Michaelis's unfortunate death as a monument to his sensitive conscience. Unfortunately I will also exhibit to the reader obstetricians whose consciences lack that of which Michaelis's had too much. May his remains rest in peace.'

We can be clear that Semmelweis too felt profoundly responsible for each and every death. Little is made, in the standard accounts, of the fact that his last professional act was to read aloud from the midwives' oath. I'm not sure what the exact words of the midwives' oath were in Budapest in 1865, but in eighteenth-century Prague the midwives' oath included an acknowledgement that the midwife would be punished with eternal damnation if any mother or infant died as a result of her ignorance. If Semmelweis read a text of this sort, then surely his last professional act was to reassert his belief that doctors were killing patients through ignorance and stupidity, and it is reasonable to conclude that his breakdown was directly caused by his sense of hopeless incapacity in the face of this situation.

It is difficult not to sympathize with Semmelweis, who certainly did know how to reduce deaths from puerperal fever. But it is also important to acknowledge that his arguments deserved to be met with puzzlement and scepticism. The original cadaverous material explanation provided a convincing account (more convincing than contemporaries were prepared to recognize) of the excess deaths on the ward where medical students were trained, but it clearly only explained a proportion of all deaths from puerperal fever. Semmelweis's revised explanation, on the other hand, provoked questions for which he had no answer.

Several critics said that if he was right, he was in effect claiming that puerperal fever was identical to the fevers that frequently killed patients who had undergone surgery. Semmelweis effectively admitted they were right (and as we have seen, Simpson had already made a connection of this sort), but he failed to follow through the logic of his argument at this point. If antiseptic measures could halt the spread of puerperal fever, then antiseptic measures could in principle be deployed to halt the spread of surgical fever: had he made this claim, Semmelweis would have pre-empted Lister. But he never made such a claim—it was as if he recognized responsibility only for obstetrical deaths. And it was natural for obstetricians to conclude that they were under no obligation to take more extensive precautions than surgeons took—which is to say, no precautions at all. It was particularly important that surgery was a much higher status discipline than the obstetrics practised in the great lying-in hospitals of the major cities, where puerperal fever was rife. Most women who came to deliver to such hospitals were unmarried, and their infants went into the foundling hospitals. As we shall see, when the surgeons discovered antiseptic principles, they were quickly adopted by obstetricians; when Semmelweis advocated the same principles it occurred neither to him nor to anyone else that the practices of the profession as a whole would have to be transformed in the light of his findings.

In addition, Semmelweis's account made puerperal fever unlike any other known disease. Many English doctors held that puerperal fever could be conveyed from one person suffering from the disease to another previously healthy woman who had recently given birth; they also suspected that those infected with erysipelas could infect others with puerperal fever. They were thus working with a model of contagion that was immediately recognizable. Semmelweis rejected this model:

> I draw different conclusions from those drawn by English physicians. I regard childbed fever as a non-contagious disease because it cannot be conveyed from every patient with childbed fever to a healthy person, and because a healthy person can contract the disease from persons not suffering from childbed fever. Every victim of smallpox is capable of giving smallpox to healthy people. A healthy person can contract smallpox only from one who has smallpox; no one has ever contracted smallpox from a person suffering from cancer of the uterus. This is not the case with childbed fever. If childbed fever takes a form in which no decaying matter is produced, then it cannot be communicated to a healthy person ... Moreover, childbed fever may come from disease states other than childbed fever, for example from gangrenous erysipelas, carcinoma of the uterus, etc. .... Every corpse, no matter what the cause of death, produces matter that can cause childbed fever.

In this debate, the English were far closer to the truth than Semmelweis. Puerperal fever is normally caused by Group A streptococcus—it is thus a contagious disease with the same cause as erysipelas. It cannot be caught, for example, from carcinoma of the uterus (unless there is a secondary infection).

The third problem with Semmelweis's theory was that he repeatedly acknowledged that the disease might be airborne. He reached this conclusion early on, in November 1847, when a patient was admitted with an infected knee. He was convinced no doctor or midwife had touched the knee, but nearly all the patients in the room died of puerperal fever. His hypothesis was that 'the icharous exhalations of the carious knee completely saturated the air of her ward'. Semmelweis was prepared to extend this admission much further than one might expect. He accepted, for example, that blocked drains could be responsible for an outbreak of puerperal fever. When in 1855 he was named Professor of Theoretical and Practical Obstetrics at the University of Pest he complained of the stale air in the clinic, of the stench from a garbage pit, and of the exhalations from the morgue: these were possible causes of puerperal fever. 'Swamp air' could easily cause an outbreak. So could overcrowding: 'If several healthy patients and their infants are in one room, the air becomes saturated with skin odours, milk secretion, lochial discharge, etc. If these exhalations are not promptly removed through ventilation they begin to decompose. If the decomposed exhalations penetrate the genitals of the patients, childbed fever can result.' Diseased patients were an even more likely source of decomposed exhalations: 'If this is what one understands by puerperal miasma, then I do not object.' At this point, Semmelweis's argument completely loses its distinctiveness, and becomes indistinguishable from miasmatic theories in general.

Semmelweis has had a peculiar place in medical history. He is lauded as a doctor who discovered how to prevent the transmission of an infectious disease, but who was ignored by his contemporaries. In a story of progress, his is an exceptional and salutary example of failure. But this is to give Semmelweis more credit than he deserves. He did not properly recognize puerperal fever as an infectious disease, or recognize the role of germs. He believed that puerperal fever could be spontaneously generated (self-infection) and that it could be transmitted by miasmas, just as his contemporaries did. He had a powerful statistical argument and a fairly effective means of prevention, but he had no account of how puerperal fever was to be compared to other fatal infections. Where Snow's arguments on the transmission of cholera were powerfully argued and virtually conclusive, Semmelweis's arguments were long-winded, puzzling, and open to obvious objections. In this book there are a number of heroic individuals who saw further than their contemporaries. Semmelweis is one of them; but his sight was no sharper than Holmes's, and his achievement far less remarkable than Snow's.

13

JOSEPH LISTER AND
ANTISEPTIC SURGERY

Modern medical science began in March 1865, when Joseph Lister, a 37-year-old professor of surgery in Glasgow, tried (unsuccessfully) to tackle a compound fracture of the leg by applying the principles of what he called 'the germ theory of putrefaction'. Compound fractures, where the broken bone sticks through the skin, were nearly always fatal prior to Lister because the wound became infected— the only remedy was amputation, which was in itself a very risky operation. Lister, like many before him, believed there was an analogy between sepsis in living tissue and putrefaction, particularly rotting meat—for one thing, the smell was the same. In the case of putrefaction it was known that tiny creatures could be seen if the flesh was inspected under a microscope; the same creatures could not be found in human pus, but it seemed plausible to imagine that this was because they were too tiny to be seen with contemporary microscopes.

Orthodox thinking was that decay was a chemical process, and that microbes were spontaneously generated as a side effect of decay. The germ theory of putrefaction claimed that the invisible living organisms were the actual cause of decay, and those invisible organisms (or their spores or germs—the term 'germ' originally refers to the dormant, infant, or seed stage of one of these invisible creatures) were wafted through the air and landed on anything and everything. Where they found suitable material their colonies flourished, feeding on biological material. The air was thus full of germs—a theory called 'panspermism'. A clear exposition of this theory had been around at least since 1799, when Spallanzani had published experiments to show 'the vast variety of animalcular eggs, scattered in the air, and falling everywhere', and the young Lister was clearly familiar with this theory (even though he was later to write as if he had never heard of germ theory before reading Pasteur), for as a young registrar in London he had persuaded himself that he could find fungal spores in gangrenous wounds. Earlier still, as a student, he had demonstrated his familiarity with the debates about spontaneous generation by getting into an argument with someone who claimed that cheese mites were spontaneously generated.

So Lister reasoned that compound fractures were fatal because germs landed on the exposed wound, and that the solution was to kill off the germs and to cover the wound. He therefore bathed the wound with carbolic acid (which had recently been introduced into the sewer system of Carlisle where it had been shown to prevent the smell of putrefaction); he cleansed the implements he used in carbolic acid; he covered the wound with dressings soaked with carbolic acid; and he placed a temporary metal plate over the whole injured area to prevent germs falling on it. He also explored methods that would make it unnecessary to reopen wounds, thus risking infection—the use of 'cat gut' (presoaked in carbolic acid, of course) for ligatures, as this was reabsorbed into the body. Later he was to advocate conducting operations while a mist of carbolic acid was being sprayed into the air, killing the germs before they could touch down, and he was to explore the use of alternative antiseptics. Although his first experiment in antiseptic surgery was a failure, his second, in August 1865, on a boy of 11 whose leg had been run over by a cart, was successful. Soon he could lay claim to a whole series of cases where his methods had saved lives, and he began publishing reports of these cases in 1867. His post-amputation death rate fell from 45 per cent to 15 per cent.

Lister's innovation was deceptively simple, and most of his own accounts of his discovery were misleading: Lister downplayed his own originality in order to win support for his new practice. In a letter to his father written in 1866, however, he said that he had made one of the ten greatest discoveries in world history, and this is perhaps to underestimate his achievement in founding medical science. The biggest advance in practical medicine before the twentieth century was Jenner's discovery of the smallpox vaccine. But what Jenner discovered was that people who had been infected with cowpox (a rare disease of cows which could be transmitted to people) never succumbed to smallpox; and he then adapted the existing programme of smallpox inoculation (which was not in itself dependent on any scientific theory, being based on folk practices common in the Middle East) by substituting cowpox inoculation, or, as he called it, vaccination (from the Latin *vacca* for cow—the term vaccination was later adopted by Pasteur to cover other forms of inoculation). Jenner had absolutely no idea of how inoculation worked or why cowpox inoculation prevented smallpox infection, and consequently his discovery did not provide the basis for further advances. Jenner was no scientist, and his account of his discovery is so straightforward that it now seems pedestrian.

In the nineteenth century brilliant physiologists such as Claude Bernard had sought to place medical knowledge on an experimental basis, through vivisection, and had discovered a great deal about human physiology. But for all their new knowledge, the new physiologists had no new therapies to offer. They were brilliant scientists, cruel men, and ineffectual doctors. With Lister, science and medicine finally meet, and medicine begins, for the first time, to save lives through the application of scientific knowledge. Lister's innovations were slow to be adopted in England (although Lister became a professor in London in 1877, few students attended his classes at first), but his methods were quickly adopted by German surgeons. In Munich post-operative mortality had been 80 per cent before the introduction of Lister's methods, and this, of course, did not include surgery on the abdomen, which was, in pre-Listerian days, almost universally fatal. Moreover his theories transformed the practice of continental obstetricians, who learnt from Lister what they had failed to learn from Semmelweis—it was Listerism that conquered puerperal fever, at least in the hospital environment. The Swiss obstetrician Johann Bischoff, for example, watched Lister at work in 1868; within a decade he had reduced puerperal fever in Basle by 80 per cent. (In some countries, England being a notable example, doctors treating mothers in their homes were very slow to adopt the necessary precautions against infection, which they dismissed as unduly time-consuming, arguing that their patients were not prepared to pay for the time involved. As a result the death rate from puerperal fever remained stubbornly high until the introduction of prontosil after 1935.)

Within a generation there was an alternative to Listerism. By 1890 Charles Lockwood was advocating aseptic or germfree rather than antiseptic or germicidal surgery. He relied on heat rather than chemicals to disinfect his implements, and water and saline rather than antiseptics to wash his patients' wounds. This was quickly to lead (in the very last years of the nineteenth century) to surgeons not only 'scrubbing' their hands before operations, but wearing rubber gloves, overalls, and face masks—Lister, by contrast, had operated wearing an old blue frockcoat, which he had previously worn in the dissecting room, and which was stiff and glazed with blood. It is worth noting that Lister had tried improved cleanliness before turning to antiseptic methods; one has to wonder whether he had the slightest idea as to how to implement such a policy. Later disagreements between the advocates of antiseptic and aseptic methods, however, should not obscure the fact that Lister had set the terms for future debate and the standard for future innovations. When Lockwood said that an operation is 'a delicate bacteriological experiment' he was restating Lister's original perception.

Lister thus begins the modern history of medicine, defined in terms of constant improvements in therapy grounded in constantly developing scientific understanding, and it is striking that it is surgery, the least theoretical of the medical disciplines, that was the first to be transformed. For all the extraordinary discoveries in bacteriology in the 1870s and 1880s, such as Koch's discovery of the anthrax bacillus in 1876, of the tuberculosis bacillus in 1882, and his (re)discovery of the cholera vibrio in 1884, the payoffs for mainstream medicine were slow to come. Pasteur discovered an anthrax vaccine in 1881, but anthrax was primarily a disease of sheep and cattle, not people. In 1885 Pasteur developed a vaccine against rabies, and although this led to an enormous expansion in research (symbolized by the founding of the Pasteur Institute), and growing confidence that diseases could be defeated by bacteriology, rabies is a very rare disease in humans. In

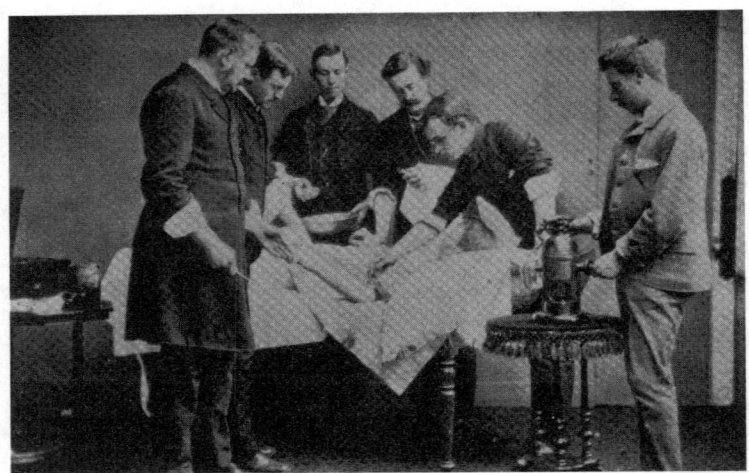

29. A surgical operation performed in Aberdeen according to Lister's principles. The pump is spraying carbolic acid. The surgeons are wearing their street clothes.

1890 Koch claimed to have identified a secret substance he called *tuberculin* that would cure tuberculosis, but he was wrong—the first effective treatment was streptomycin, discovered in 1944. In 1892 Haffkine finally developed a vaccine against cholera, but in Europe at least cholera had been almost eliminated; in 1897 Almroth Wright (in whose laboratory Fleming was later to 'discover' penicillin) developed a vaccine against typhoid, but typhoid was primarily a disease of the tropics and (during the First World War) the trenches. From 1876 (Koch's discovery of the anthrax bacillus) until 1894 the triumphs of germ theory, and triumphs they were, were confined to surgery, army medicine, and tropical medicine. But in 1894 the Pasteur Institute discovered a bacteriological diagnosis and treatment for diphtheria, a disease that was very widespread in temperate climates and sometimes fatal.

This treatment consisted in injecting blood serum from an animal which had acquired immunity to diphtheria into a human being who had recently been infected but lacked immunity—it was thus very different from a vaccine, which makes the patient immune through a controlled infection. Diphtheria was the first specific infection to be successfully treated in general medical practice, and therefore the decisive moment when germ theory entered mainstream medicine and began to transform the education and the practice of ordinary doctors in the developed world. It came almost thirty years after Lister's revolution in surgery. Nevertheless, if the new bacteriology took time to come up with cures to prevalent diseases, and if it was defeated by killers such as TB, progress was steady and cumulative. Obstacles were overcome and solutions found. The confident claims of the new bacteriology's supporters were certainly premature—in 1876 John Tyndall had claimed that epidemic diseases would soon be swept from the face of the earth—but they were not entirely misplaced. This is a story of good medicine, and it belongs in a different book.

In the conventional story, the triumph of germ theory begins with Koch's discovery of the anthrax bacillus and ends with Wright's conquest of typhoid. This story is a story of technique: Koch's use of solid (gelatine, agar) rather than liquid mediums for the cultivation of pure samples of bacteria, and the invention of the petri dish; the invention of methods of dyeing bacteria to make them visible under the microscope; Pasteur's triumph in learning how to attenuate or weaken anthrax bacteria so that they could safely be injected into cows and sheep. In this story, Lister disappears into germ theory's prehistory, and is merely 'the English disciple' of Pasteur, a role in which, it must be said, he cast himself. As a result, the nature of the first crucial meeting between science and medicine is scarcely explored and its character is systematically misunderstood.

Modern history of science, including history of medicine, has consistently sought to destroy the notion that there is a straightforward logic of discovery: that one discovery leads almost automatically to another, that one researcher picks up where another has left off, as if passing a baton in a relay race. At stake is Pasteur's claim that scientific research pursues an 'inflexible logic'. Instead recent histories insist that there are always conflicting views, uncertain outcomes, unpredictable developments. Lister said he was applying 'germ

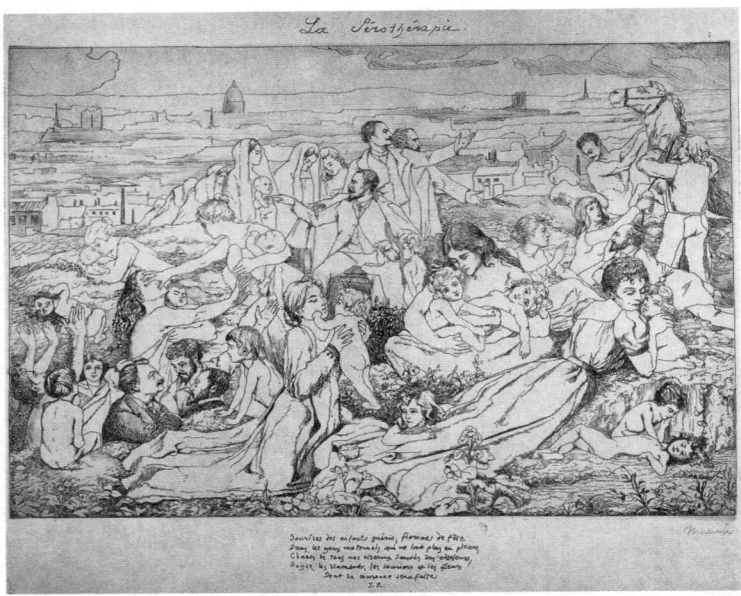

30. This etching by Charles Maurin, *c.* 1896, shows the researchers from the Institut Pasteur, led by Pierre-Paul-Emil Roux, who had discovered serum therapy for diphtheria. On the right is the horse from whose blood the serum comes. The poem, by Jean Richepin, is translated by Suzanne G. Lindsay as: 'Smiles of children cured, / Festive sparks in the mothers' eyes that weep no more, / Songs of all our birds saved from the birdcatchers, / Be the diamonds, the laurels, and the flowers of which his crown will be made.'

theory' to the most intractable problem in surgery; in a characteristic move, the latest book on the subject, says that there were always numerous 'germ theories', not one germ theory, and indeed that Lister's own stated views on germs changed significantly over time. And this is correct: Lister, who started out claiming that one needed to accept the truth of germ theory in order to successfully implement his practices, quickly retreated to saying that he did not care what people believed as long as they did what he said. But in 1865 Pasteur was the only germ theorist of note, so that germ theory, when Lister first introduced antiseptic surgery, was nothing other than Pasteur's germ theory, and Lister always uses the term in the singular, as when he said in 1875 that 'the philosophical investigations of Pasteur long since made me a convert to the germ theory'. It is also said that at first Lister's germs 'were more like seeds of disease, highly plastic agents (not specific causal entities) whose pathogenic qualities depended on the local environment in which they developed'.

Lister's germ theory is thus presented as primitive and unsophisticated. But while this may be true of some germ theories of the 1870s and 1880s, it is not true of Lister's. What Lister meant (at least in his early work) by 'germ theory' was quite specifically the germ theory of putrefaction. He was quite clear that 'the character of the decomposition which occurs in a given fermentable substance is determined by the nature of the organism that develops in it', which is a way of saying that germs are specific causal entities. It would be wrong to identify his public statements (which were aimed at winning support for antiseptic surgery in the face of bitter opposition) with his private commitments. And yet for all these (often misguided) attempts to read Lister on the assumption that he was not a modern germ theorist, every book reproduces as established fact a false impression carefully conveyed by Lister's first publication: that Lister's success was entirely dependent on his reading of Pasteur, and in particular of Pasteur's famous publications of 1861–2 on spontaneous generation. In all his early papers, we are told, Lister 'cited Pasteur's germ theory as his inspiration'. Three years, we are to understand, was all that it took for Pasteur's work to have a decisive impact on medical practice. The baton was passed from Pasteur to Lister and has never been dropped since.

But Lister's own most detailed account of his discovery is difficult to reconcile with this conventional story that appears to be so firmly grounded in Lister's own words. And once we consider Lister's own assessment of the preconditions for his discovery we are bound to realize that progress in medicine has been even more puzzling and problematic than historians of science have been prepared to recognize. Even when at their most sceptical they have been seduced by a fairy tale constructed by Lister to charm his readers.

According to Lister's first publication on the antiseptic method, which appeared in 1867, if we ask

> how the atmosphere produces decomposition of organic substances, we find that a flood of light has been thrown upon this most important subject by the philosophic researches of Pasteur, who has demonstrated by thoroughly convincing evidence that it is not to its oxygen or to any of its gaseous constituents that the air owes this property, but to minute particles suspended in it, which are the germs of various low forms of life, long since revealed by microscope, and regarded as merely accidental concomitants of putrescence, but now shown by Pasteur to be its essential cause . . .

And he then says that 'a beautiful illustration of this doctrine' is presented by cases where a lung is punctured by a fractured rib. Here, though air enters the lung, no infection ever occurs, whereas if there is an external opening in the chest infection always takes place. And this Lister reasons is because the atmospheric gases entering the lung have been filtered in their passage through the bronchial tubes. In operations one needs to create a germfree environment such as exists within the lung. How to do this? 'In the course of the year 1864 I was much struck with an account of the remarkable effects produced by carbolic acid upon the sewage of the town of Carlisle . . .' And so the antiseptic system was born. The story seems straightforward; first Pasteur, then reflection on punctured lungs, then carbolic acid. And this is the story told by historians.

But it is plain wrong. In 1868 Lister described in detail, in a lecture delivered in Glasgow, Pasteur's famous experiments on whose authority he had relied the year before, followed by some experiments of his own along the same lines. And then he says: 'This mode of experimenting, as described by Pasteur, besides charming me by its simplicity and conclusiveness, had a further special interest for myself, because, *before knowing of it* [my italics], I had explained to my own mind on the same principle the remarkable fact, previously quite inexplicable' that infection does not follow when a lung is punctured by a fractured rib. He had begun to think about this problem, he tells us, thirteen years before (i.e.

*c.*1855) when he had conducted an autopsy on someone with a punctured lung.

> Why air introduced into the pleura through a wounded lung should have such totally different effects from that entering through a permanently open penetrating wound from without, was to me a complete mystery till I heard of the germ theory of putrefaction, when it at once occurred to me that, though we could not suppose the gases of the atmosphere to be in any way altered in chemical composition by passing through the trachea and bronchial tubes on their way into the pleura, it was only natural that they should be filtered of germs by the air-passages, one of whose offices is to arrest inhaled particles of dust, and prevent them from entering the air-cells. In truth, this fact in practical surgery, when duly considered, affords as good evidence in support of the germ theory of putrefaction as any experiment that can be performed artificially.

It so happens that Lister himself tells us that he became interested in carbolic acid in 1864, and first read Pasteur (on the recommendation of his colleague, Thomas Anderson) in 1865. The real chronology thus appears to be as follows:

1855: Lister discovers the problem of the punctured but uninfected lung.

1860–4: Lister solves this problem on hearing of the germ theory of putrefaction, but before he has read Pasteur. (Lister had arrived in Glasgow in 1860 satisfied that exposure to oxygen was the cause of putrefaction, so he did not have the solution then.)

1864: He realizes that carbolic acid would make a suitable antiseptic.

March 1865: He conducts the first antiseptic operation.

Sometime in 1865 he reads Pasteur.

1867: he presents his new practice as if it had been inspired by reading Pasteur.

We thus face a simple question: Where did Lister first encounter the germ theory of putrefaction? There are two possibilities here. One is that Lister's account is intended to separate his hearing of

Pasteur's work in his conversation with Anderson from his first reading Pasteur. On this interpretation, Lister's breakthrough did not require any detailed knowledge of Pasteur's experiments. The other is that he first encountered germ theory by a quite different route.

No one was better placed to learn about germ theory than Lister. His father, Joseph Jackson Lister, an amateur naturalist, had solved the problem of chromatic distortion in compound microscopes, both in theory (it had long been thought insoluble) and in practice, and in the 1830s, when Lister was a youth, his father was producing the finest microscopes the world had ever seen. Lister's first scientific publication, in 1853, on the structure of the iris, was in the *Quarterly Journal of Microscopical Science*. His most important early work, published in the *Transactions of the Royal Society* in 1858, dealt with inflammation, blood coagulation, and the electrical stimulation of nerves, and relied on vivisection and microscopic inspection. From this work it is clear that Lister was reading the current literature in Latin, French, and German.

Pasteur's famous series of papers in 1862 reported a series of experiments designed to refute the claims of Felix-Archimède Pouchet, who claimed to have demonstrated spontaneous generation. Pasteur filtered air and found microscopic creatures in it. He sterilized sugared yeast-water liquid by boiling it for a few minutes and placed it in flasks containing air that had been heated by a red-hot platinum tube: no putrefaction took place. He briefly exposed sterilized liquids prone to fermentation to the atmosphere in different places—at the top of a mountain, on a glacier, in the vaults of the Paris observatory, on the busy rue d'Ulm in Paris—and then sealed them again, and was able to show that different atmospheres carried infective agents in different degrees. He placed both sterilized and unsterilized liquids in flasks with wavy swan-necks—the sterilized liquids did not ferment, even though the flasks were open to the exterior atmosphere, because the micro-organisms in the atmosphere were trapped in the swan-necks and never reached the body of the flask. This was the experiment—devised not by Pasteur but by Michel Chevreul, and first published by Pasteur—that delighted Lister in 1865 and that he repeated with modifications in 1868: Pasteur's swan-necked flasks modelled exactly the function attributed by Lister to the trachea and bronchial tubes in cases where a fractured rib had punctured a lung.

One group of experiments performed by Pasteur, where both his liquids and the air in his flasks were sterilized by heat, were essentially repetitions of a well-known set of experiments reported by Theodore Schwann in 1837. Schwann had started by repeating Spallanzani's experiments which had involved heating liquids in sealed vessels, but it could be argued that putrefaction failed to take place afterwards because some change had taken place in the quality of the air as a result of heating in the presence of (in this case) a meat broth, that there was, for example, no longer any oxygen available to sustain life. So Schwann devised flasks that were open to the atmosphere, but, once the liquid in them had been boiled, air could only enter after being heated 'almost to the boiling point of mercury' (357° C). No

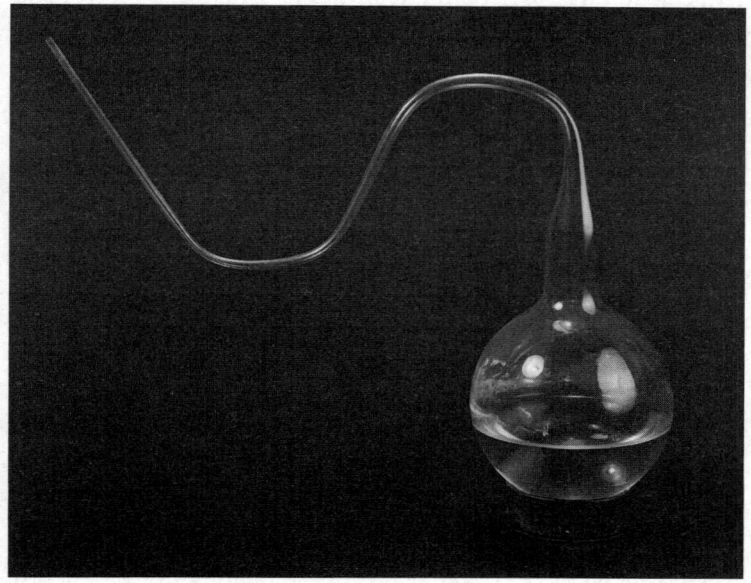

31. Swan-necked flask used by Pasteur in his experiments to disprove spontaneous generation.

life developed in these flasks, although they certainly contained oxygen: Schwann took this to be a decisive blow to theories of spontaneous generation.

Schwann's experiments differed from Pasteur's in a number of key respects: Schwann studied first putrefaction and then fermentation, while Pasteur studied first fermentation and then (publishing in 1863) putrefaction. Although the two processes were recognized to be comparable, when Lister repeated Pasteur's early experiments in 1867 he substituted urine for Pasteur's sugar and yeast in order to confirm his results for putrefaction. But Schwann had gone on to try and identify what sort of microscopic creatures he was dealing with by trying various poisons on them: putrefaction, he thought he could show, was caused by both invisible animals and invisible plants, while fermentation was caused only by invisible plants. Schwann's experiments were important because they appeared to show that alcoholic fermentation was not a chemical process in the presence of a catalyst (as was generally thought) but a biological process: Pasteur was to develop this line of argument in 1857 in an important paper on lactic fermentation.

If we look at Schwann's work it is immediately obvious that it is as close as Pasteur's to the 'bacteriological experiment' involved in Lister's antiseptic surgery: both studied putrefaction, but it was Schwann who tried to halt the process of putrefaction. Pasteur hypothesized that if you were to wrap a piece of meat in a cloth moistened with alcohol and then seal it in a jar putrefaction would not occur, but Schwann experimented with particular antiseptic agents. We might say that Schwann's experimental work was entirely germicidal, because it took panspermism for granted, while Pasteur had shown that in the mountain air of a glacier or in a swan-necked vase one could find an effectively germfree environment. In this respect Lister's work derives directly from Schwann's line of thinking, while Lockwood's derives from Pasteur's.

When Lister told his Glasgow audience in 1868 that he had worked out his theory of antiseptic surgery as soon as he had learnt of the germ theory of putrefaction, and before he had read Pasteur's work, we must recognize the possibility that at some time between

1860 (when he arrived in Glasgow) and 1864 (when he began to consider the possible applications of carbolic acid), Lister had become familiar with Schwann's work, and seen that it provided an answer to the puzzling failure of putrefaction to develop in lungs punctured by broken ribs: the air within the lungs had been filtered of germs. Schwann's work with poisons pointed directly to the possibility of antiseptic surgery, but the poison he had used to prevent putrefaction was arsenic, which could not be applied to surgical wounds without endangering the patient. Further progress thus depended on Lister learning of a poison that was fatal to germs but could be tolerated by humans—on learning of the use of carbolic acid in sewers in 1864 he knew everything he needed to know. Lister did not need any knowledge of Pasteur's work to develop antiseptic surgery.

This is more or less what he tells us himself, although historians, mesmerized by the notion that Pasteur's work was of fundamental importance, have been quite incapable of hearing what Lister says. In 1869 Lister became professor of surgery in Edinburgh, and delivered there a lecture which was not initially intended for publication. In it he described how:

> The first great step towards the establishment of this theory [*the germ theory of putrefaction*] was the discovery of the yeast plant in 1838 by Cagniard-Latour . . . In the following year, Schwann of Berlin published the results of a remarkable investigation into the cause of putrefaction (in the course of which, by a coincidence such as is not uncommon in the history of science, he too had independently discovered the yeast plant), and he related experiments which showed that a decoction of meat might remain for weeks together free alike from putrefaction and from the development of infusoria or fungi in a flask containing air frequently renewed, provided that the atmosphere was subjected to a high temperature at some part of its course towards the containing vessel. Hence he concluded that putrefaction was caused by the growth of organisms springing from germs in the air, the heat preventing the putrefactive change by depriving the germs of their vitality. In other words, he propounded the germ theory of putrefaction. . . . Schwann's observations, however, did not receive the attention which they appear to me to have deserved.

Thus if Lister did not learn of the germ theory of putrefaction by reading Schwann (and this seems to me a real possibility), then he certainly knew by 1869 that all he needed to know to develop antiseptic surgery could have been learnt from Schwann.

Yet Lister continued to praise Pasteur as if he alone was responsible for the germ theory of putrefaction. Why? There is, I think, an obvious answer to this question. Schwann's work had always been controversial. The leading chemist of the day, von Liebig, had rejected it, and efforts to reproduce his experiments had been unsuccessful—'It is true, indeed,' Lister said in 1869 of Schwann's work, 'that if you attempt to repeat the experiments you may meet with failure.' Pasteur's work on the other hand was not only new and fashionable—it had been discussed, for example, by Thomas Wells in an address to the BMA in August 1864—but Pasteur's work had been ratified, as Lister stressed, 'by the report of the Commission of the French Academy', first in 1862 and then in 1864. Pasteur was an authority on whom he could safely rely—or at least so he seemed until Bastian claimed once again to be able to demonstrate spontaneous generation.

Does it matter whether Pasteur's research was crucial to Lister's innovation in surgery? It matters a great deal. If it was, Lister can be safely accommodated within the relay-race model of medical progress. Pasteur, Lister, Koch, Pasteur, Wright—the baton was passed from one to the other without being dropped. In this list, Lister seems the least important, because he merely found a new practical application for Pasteur's work on spontaneous generation. But if Schwann's work could equally have inspired Lister, then a yawning gap opens up. Schwann's work had been published in 1837 (not 1839, as Lister thought), and Lister did not publish until 1867. For thirty years the intellectual principles required for antiseptic surgery had been widely known and much discussed, but no one grasped their possible application. Carbolic acid was, it is true, a missing piece of the jigsaw, but Lister quickly discovered that there were a number of suitable alternative antiseptics, and (as Pasteur had claimed) even alcohol would have done perfectly well. Pasteur's own paper had referred to the work of Pringle, published in 1752, which had concluded that there were numerous antiseptics. There was no inherent difficulty in finding a suitable antiseptic once one started looking for it.

It is time to complete the quotation from Tyndall that serves as an epigraph to this book:

> It is interesting and indeed pathetic to observe how long a discovery of priceless value to humanity may be hidden away, or rather lie openly revealed, before the final and apparently obvious step is taken towards its practical application. In 1837, Schwann clearly established the connection between putrefaction and microscopic life; but thirty years had to elapse before Lister extended to wounds the researches of Schwann on dead flesh and animal infusions.

The real measure of nineteenth-century medical science is not the three-year gap between Pasteur being awarded the prize of the French Academy for disproving spontaneous generation and Lister's first operation, but the thirty-year gap between Schwann's work and Lister's. The size of this gap makes very plain the important fact that there was nothing obvious or routine about turning the new principles of bacteriology into new medical practices—Lister's work is hopelessly underestimated if one takes at face value his own unduly modest suggestion that it followed straightforwardly from reading Pasteur. To make the leap that Lister made you needed to be a microscopist (to have seen all the invisible creatures in the air), a bacteriologist (to understand that every operation was a bacteriological experiment), and a surgeon, accustomed to struggling with sepsis. In the thirty years since the publication of Schwann's work, Lister may have been the first person to meet all three requirements, which partially explains the long delay. It also helped that Lister was surrounded by people who were worrying about the spread of infections in hospital wards: since Lister believed that diseases were spread not by miasmas, but by germs floating through the air, the covering of wounds with antiseptic dressings was, he was convinced, enough to prevent infections spreading from patient to patient—as a result he claimed to have eliminated pyemia, hospital gangrene, and erysipelas from his wards, despite the fact that the air was as foul and smelly as always (which was attributed to the fact that the Glasgow Infirmary had been built over the graves of the cholera victims of 1849 and next to the Cathedral churchyard). Indeed Lister even took pride in the fact that his wards were cleaned less often than most hospital wards: once he knew that it was germs that were the enemy, smells and even ordinary dirt ceased to worry him.

But at the same time it is clear that for at least thirty years patients had been dying unnecessarily. The key intellectual preconditions for antiseptic surgery had been met by 1837; indeed Schwann was only belatedly developing the work of Spallanzani, who was only belatedly following up on the ideas of Leeuwenhoek. The key obstacle to medical progress was not intellectual but cultural: the best doctors and the best scientists failed to acknowledge the importance of the microscope, and they changed their minds only as it became apparent (though it should have been apparent from the beginning) that neither traditional views on disease, nor the new chemical theories could produce effective remedies.

The genius of Pasteur was to make an early commitment to the idea that processes standardly thought to be chemical were in fact biological, and then, in the light of this commitment, to tackle one problem after another: first the fermentation of alcohol (1857–65), then silkworm diseases (1865–70), then anthrax (1877–81), and finally rabies (1880–4). Pasteur crept up on medicine because the obstacles there were greater: in the case of silkworm diseases, all that was necessary was to establish which silkworms were infected and kill them; similar principles could hardly be applied to humans. He also had a perfectly sensible distrust of doctors: he was reluctant to work with them, and found them resistant to progress. Lister, by contrast, applied the new science directly to medicine from the beginning (although he also carried out numerous vivisections); he did his best to carry the medical profession with him, and had considerable success. Suppose Leeuwenhoek had had a second and a third generation of pupils, instead of being left without any successors. Could there have been an early eighteenth-century Pasteur? Surely not. Enormous advances in chemistry were a precondition for Pasteur's work. But why should there not have been an early eighteenth-century Lister? Is there anything in Lister's key articles that he could not have explained and made comprehensible to Leeuwenhoek? Is there anything that

Leeuwenhoek would have thought was not a natural development from his own work? The answer to these questions, I think, has to be no, and the implication is that there can be no satisfactory intellectual history of medicine between 1677 and 1867, for the real question is not 'What discoveries made it possible for medicine to develop as it did?' But 'What psychological, cultural, or institutional factors represented an obstacle to medicine developing as it might have?' I will try to answer this question in the conclusion to this Part.

14

ALEXANDER FLEMING
AND PENICILLIN

In September 1928 Alexander Fleming returned from holiday and began to sort through the mess in his laboratory. At first he discarded a culture plate that had been lying in the open air for some weeks. On it a blob of mould had interfered with the development of the staphylococci that had been sown on the jellied broth. Glancing at it again, Fleming rescued the plate from the bath of disinfectant in which it was about to be immersed. Six years earlier he had discovered a substance called lysozyme, a substance found in tears, saliva, and mucus, which had shown a similar capacity to kill off bacteria. Lysozyme, it had turned out, had little effect on those bacteria that cause dangerous diseases, but Fleming's experience with it meant he only needed a glance at his contaminated plate to recognize that something important might be happening, for on this plate the unknown mould was killing an organism which was a common source of dangerous infections, a staphylococcus.

It was straightforward to establish that the mould was a member of the *Penicillium* family, and that it was active against numerous dangerous bacteria. Fleming could easily show that it did no harm to white blood cells: this was important because the laboratory he worked in, headed by Almroth Wright, had long been committed to the idea that the key to effective treatment was to mobilize the body's own capacity for defence. Fleming himself, during the First World War, had studied infections in soldiers' wounds and had argued that conventional antiseptics both killed off white blood cells faster than they killed bacteria, and failed to penetrate into the jagged interstices of gunshot wounds: they were, he thought, positively fostering infection.

He could also straightforwardly show, by injecting the broth derived from his mould into a very small number of mice and rabbits, that it was not toxic. And he could also show that it quickly lost its antibacterial effect when mixed with digestive juices: there would be no point in taking it as a pill.

Fleming was surely moving towards injecting penicillin (as he was soon to call his 'mould broth filtrate') into infected animals to see if it would cure them. He had long worked with salvarsan, which was the first drug effective against syphilis, a disease that Fleming had extensive experience of treating in private practice. But by April 1929 he seems to have lost all interest in injecting penicillin into the bloodstream. Penicillin took around four hours to kill bacteria; but tests showed that both in animals and in the test tube it ceased to be active in blood after two hours. This seems to have persuaded him that it would be pointless introducing penicillin into a diseased body.

This left the alternative of applying penicillin topically to local infections. He used it successfully on a case of conjunctivitis, and applied it to carbuncles with mixed results. An attempt to treat a case of septicaemia was a failure. The possibility that penicillin might have a future use as an antiseptic was mentioned in Fleming's first and only major publication on his new discovery, which appeared in 1929. He wrote: 'It is suggested that it may be an efficient antiseptic for application to, or injection into, areas infected with penicillin-sensitive microbes.' But between 1930 and 1940 Fleming made no effort to develop a clinical use for penicillin. Throughout this period, however, he employed it regularly for the one use that was outlined in his key publication. While penicillin killed many bacteria, it did not kill a bacterium called Pfeiffer's bacterium, which some (including Fleming) thought might be the main cause of influenza. Pfeiffer's bacterium was very difficult to cultivate because it was usually contaminated by other bacteria that grew more vigorously and overwhelmed it. Fleming found that if he took a sample of mucus and spread it over a petri dish treated with penicillin, then he could grow a pure sample of Pfeiffer's bacterium, because it was immune to penicillin, while the bacteria that normally overwhelmed it were sensitive to it.

Fleming was happy with this discovery because the laboratory in which he worked was funded by the production of vaccines. Almroth Wright in effect ran a private company within St Mary's Hospital in London; from its income he ran a couple of wards and paid the salaries of a small staff. The enterprise seems also to have been personally profitable for Wright and his close associates, including Fleming. Wright had discovered the vaccine against typhoid, a conventional prophylactic vaccine, but from his starting work at St Mary's in 1902 until his retirement in 1946 his main preoccupation was producing vaccines that would be given to people after they had become infected and would stimulate the body's defences—the model was Pasteur's vaccine against rabies, which was injected after the victim had been bitten by a rabid dog. Wright and Fleming (Fleming had charge of the production of vaccines from 1920 on) produced vaccines against acne, boils, influenza, gonorrhoea, tuberculosis, and cancer. The modern view would be that all these vaccines were totally ineffectual: the whole profitable business was founded on a failure to carry out adequate controlled trials to see if people receiving Wright's vaccines did better than those not receiving them. Wright had been involved in a controversy over the statistics he had used to show that his typhoid vaccine (which really was effective) worked, and he carefully avoided subjecting his new vaccines to proper tests. Instead he invented a spurious measure, the opsonin index, of the body's resistance to infection, and claimed this measured the improvement resulting from his vaccinations. Fleming thus made a very good living out of selling what were, in effect, sophisticated quack remedies. Penicillin, he hoped, would enable him to produce an 'improved' influenza vaccine.

Although Fleming recognized that penicillin might possibly have a therapeutic use, he was far too interested in the production of vaccines to waste much time exploring the possibility. A few discouraging findings, and he dropped all work on it. He was also quite uninterested in the problem of how to produce purer, stronger samples of his new drug. Two students of his, Ridley and Craddock, did astonishingly able work, under horribly primitive conditions (they worked on tables in a corridor, and had to go to the next floor to find running water), to produce a purer drug. They evaporated a broth made from the penicillin under a vacuum, and dissolved the penicillin in alcohol, in the process purifying it further. Where their first preparations were highly unstable, they discovered that they could make the penicillin stable by adding acid. Fleming seems to have had virtually no interest in their work. He misreported some of their findings in his first publication, and later claimed that the problem of producing stable penicillin had proved insoluble. When others set about producing penicillin in a purer and more stable form, they had to rediscover everything that Ridley and Craddock had discovered because Fleming never mentioned their work to later investigators. Fleming himself was quite happy using the impure penicillin broth, which was perfectly adequate for the production of uncontaminated samples of Pfeiffer's bacillus.

In September 1939 (to be exact on 6 September, three days after the declaration of war), eleven years after Fleming's discovery, Howard Florey, in Oxford, began to seek funding for penicillin research—for a year or so his colleague Ernst Chain had been cultivating penicillin derived from Fleming's original strain. Florey and Chain were engaged in a systematic search to find biological agents (rather than the chemical agents already developed into salvarsan and prontosil) which would be capable of killing the bacteria that caused fatal infections, and penicillin was only one agent on their shortlist of promising substances. In May 1940 they had enough purified penicillin to carry out a straightforward experiment: injecting penicillin into four mice that had been infected with streptococci—four others were infected but not given penicillin. The results were dramatic, for the mice treated with penicillin survived in good health, and those not treated died. They were confirmed when the experiment was repeated the next day. From the first, the Oxford team (two professors and seven researchers) were convinced they had a discovery of the foremost importance—they smeared the spores of Fleming's strain of penicillin into the linings of their coats, so that if the Germans invaded they could preserve their raw material.

In August 1940 they published the results of their animal experiments; a year later they published the results of the first trials on humans, although the quantities of penicillin available meant that it had been possible to treat only five patients. All had shown astonishing improvements, although two had died. The most striking case, perhaps, was the cure of a boy of 14 with staphylococcal septicaemia from an osteomyelitis of the left femur, a condition previously almost invariably fatal. In August 1941 the results of these trials were published, and the race was on to produce penicillin in commercial quantities. By June 1943, penicillin production in the US was enough to treat 170 cases a month; a year later it was enough to treat 40,000 cases a month, or all the battlefield casualties of the Allied invasion of Europe; and within another year it was enough to treat a quarter of a million patients a month. That year, 1945, Fleming, Florey and Chain shared the Nobel prize for medicine. A medical revolution had taken place within the space of four years.

From the beginning, Fleming and his associates sought to claim for him the credit for the therapeutic use of penicillin. In September 1940, after the publication of Florey and Chain's animal experiments, Fleming himself wrote to the *British Medical Journal* pointing out that he had foreseen a therapeutic use in his 1929 paper. In September 1941, after the publication of the first clinical trials, Almroth Wright wrote to *The Times* (which had published a leading article on penicillin) to claim the credit for the discovery for Fleming. Fleming, who had abandoned work on the clinical use of penicillin within months of his first discovery, happily answered calls from the press. He rapidly became famous throughout the world as the discoverer of penicillin, while Florey and Chain were left in obscurity. Fleming's contribution only began to be placed in proper perspective with the publication of Ronald Hare's *The Birth of Penicillin* in 1970.

The story I have just told is now a familiar one. It was Florey and Chain, not Fleming, who demonstrated the clinical value of penicillin, and they and their associates who began to solve the problems of producing penicillin on an industrial scale. But their key experiment of May 1940 could have been carried out by Fleming, who certainly had, particularly as a result of the unappreciated work of Ridley and Craddock, an adequate supply of penicillin to inject into mice. Had he done this experiment in 1929 literally millions of lives could have been saved, lives that were lost without an adequate broad-spectrum antibiotic. (Some writers have claimed that the technology of freeze-drying was essential for the Oxford work, and was not available in 1929; but Ridley and Craddock's work shows that Fleming could have managed without it.) If Fleming deserves the credit for recognizing the action of penicillin on his contaminated dish, he also carries the responsibility for this delay.

The situation would thus appear straightforward: Fleming discovered penicillin; Florey and Chain first put it to effective use. The question of the relative contribution of Fleming on the one hand, and Florey and Chain on the other to the revolution represented by modern drug therapy has however distracted attention from an even more puzzling and difficult question. In what sense can Fleming be said to have discovered penicillin?

Contamination of bacterial cultures by moulds takes place all the time. In 1871 Sir John Burdon Sanderson reported that moulds of the *Penicillium* group would prevent the development of bacteria in a broth exposed to the air. In 1872 Joseph Lister established that the growth of *Penicillium glaucum* would kill off bacteria in a liquid culture. He at once saw the possible clinical application of the phenomenon. He wrote to his brother saying 'Should a suitable case present, I shall endeavour to employ *Penicillium glaucum* and observe if the growth of the organisms be inhibited in the human tissues.' He never published his results, so we do not know how far and how long he pursued the question, but we do know that in 1884 a patient of Lister's, a young nurse, was suffering from an infected wound. Various chemical antiseptics were tried without success, and then a new substance was used. She was so astonished and so grateful at her seemingly miraculous cure that she asked Lister's registrar to write the name of this substance in her scrap-book. It was *penicillium*. Why did Lister keep this success to himself? There is, I think, only one possible explanation. Throughout the 1870s and 1880s he was struggling to win acceptance for the principle of antiseptic surgery. He lacked the energy or the resources to embark on a new campaign while the germ theory itself remained so widely contested.

In 1895 Vincenzo Tiberio in Naples injected extracts of *penicillium* moulds into infected animals, the experiment 'first' performed by Florey and Chain in 1940, though his results were nothing like as striking as theirs. In 1897, a young French army doctor called Duchesne described similar experiments in a thesis. His preliminary results were certainly striking; unfortunately he died of tuberculosis before he could carry out further trials. Fleming was blissfully ignorant of all this previous work. Had he known of it he might have been less quick to claim the credit for the discovery of a new substance.

Gwyn MacFarlane, whose fine book on Fleming is my source for this information, tries to play down its significance. He argues that the mould Fleming discovered in 1929 was a rare strain of *Penicillium notatum*. Where many strains of *penicillium* are completely inactive, including most strains of *Penicillium notatum*, Fleming's strain was peculiarly powerful. Exhaustive studies in the early 1940s were to find only two more powerful strains among hundreds tested.

> Fleming's rare strain of P. notatum was far more active than any used by Burdon-Sanderson, Lister, Tiberio, Duchesne, and many others from 1870 onwards. If any one of these had been lucky enough to have been visited by the mould that alighted on Fleming's plate in 1928, they too would have discovered penicillin and might possibly have taken it further than he did . . .

Here Macfarlane states as a fact what is at best a statement of probability. We do not know exactly what strains Burdon Sanderson, Lister, Tiberio, Duchesne and the others worked with. We do know however that none of them had difficulty finding active strains of *penicillium*, and that in every case the activity of the *penicillium* was sufficiently marked to suggest that it had clinical potential. Others too watched *penicillium* killing off bacteria. Tyndall, for example, had noted in test tube after test tube 'the struggle for existence between the *Bacteria* and the *Penicillium*', although he had not grasped the potential significance of what his eyes had seen. Thus it would seem fair to say that Lister and Duchesne had both independently discovered penicillin, and had taken it somewhat further than Fleming did, and that there was nothing remarkable in Fleming's initial identification of *penicillium* as an antibiotic.

Moreover the idea behind the research project of Florey and Chain, the idea that one could find biological agents capable of killing off infectious diseases (what we now call antibiotics), was not a new one. Lister had immediately recognized the potential of *penicillium* in 1872. Arnaldo Cantani had used bacteria painted on the throat of a sick child to reduce her fever in 1885, and had stated the principles involved. So the larger project envisaged by Florey and Chain, that of research on what was initially called bacterial antagonism, was not original—one of the major purposes of a book published by George Papacostas and Jean Gaté in 1928, *Les Associations microbiennes*, was to collect together in one place the information on this. Here again we encounter the same phenomenon that we have encountered so often before. The true puzzle about penicillin is why it was not brought into medical use fifty years earlier. Florey and Chain discovered an effective antibiotic within months of starting looking for one; there is no reason to think that a similar achievement was beyond a Pasteur or a Lister.

CONCLUSION TO PART III: PROGRESS DELAYED

In 1879 an American doctor, T. H. Buckler acknowledged that 'the lancet, by the common consent of the profession at large, had been sheathed never to be drawn again'. Yet he was writing 'A Plea for the Lancet'. In 1875 an English doctor, W. Mitchell Clarke, wrote 'we are most decidedly living in one of the periods when the lancet is carried idly in its silver case; no one bleeds; and yet from the way in which I find my friends retain their lancets, and keep them from rusting, I cannot help thinking they look forward to a time when they will employ them again'. Bloodletting had largely been abandoned because statistical studies had shown that it did not work, and recent developments in physiology had been able to show that it resulted in reduced haemoglobin concentration, which hardly seemed likely to be beneficial. But doctors clearly regretted sheathing their lancets. The lancet was the symbol of their profession and of their status as doctors—the leading English medical journal is still called *The Lancet*.

Worst of all though, the abandonment of the lancet was not compensated for by the introduction of any new therapy that could replace it in general practice. A gap was left, and something was needed to fill the gap. By 1892 the leading American physician of his day, William Osler, was writing 'During the first five decades of this century the profession bled too much, but during the last decades we have certainly bled too little.' And he proceeded to advocate blood-letting for pneumonia: done early it could 'save life'. Similarly in 1903 Robert Reyburn, an American, was asking 'Have we not lost something of value to our science in our entire abandonment of the practice of venesection?' *The Lancet* of 1911 contained an article entitled 'Cases illustrating the uses of venesection'—the cases included high blood pressure and cerebral haemorrhage. Bloodletting was also recommended for various types of poisoning, from carbon monoxide to mustard gas. In the trenches in 1916, venesection was the approved method of treating the victims of gas attacks. Heinrich Stern, publishing *The Theory and Practice of Bloodletting* in New York in 1915 declared that 'like a phoenix, the fabulous bird, bloodletting has outlasted the centuries and has risen, rejuvenated, and with new vigor, from the ashes of fire which threatened its destruction'—he thought bloodletting a useful treatment for drunkenness and homosexuality. Others recommended it for typhoid, influenza, jaundice, arthritis, eczema, and epilepsy.

At the beginning of this book, I said that 1865 was a useful marker, but that medicine was not at once transformed. Just as new, effective therapies were only developed slowly in the years after 1865, so old therapies were only slowly phased out. Hippocratic therapies survived into the 1920s. Why was progress so slow? It was not because doctors like Osler were opposed to modern science, or did not believe in the idea of progress; quite the contrary. We need to look elsewhere for an explanation. Part of the explanation lies in the way in which people identify with their own skills, particularly when they have gone to great trouble and expense to acquire them. Just as surgeons wanted to go on being surgeons, and so were blind to the possibilities of anaesthetics, so doctors wanted to go on being doctors, and so were reluctant to sheath their lancets.

Another part of the explanation lies in the risk associated with pursuing new ideas. Once germ theory had begun to establish itself, people like Tyndall were convinced that contagious disease could be conquered. But there existed only one model for the defeat of a contagious disease, and that was smallpox vaccination. So most of the effort went into the pursuit of vaccines: anthrax, rabies, and typhoid vaccines were the result. Germ theory could equally have rapidly led to a search for substances that could be injected into the bloodstream to kill germs. Penicillin could have been developed at almost any point after 1872. But there was no conceptual model for an antibiotic. The risks seemed high and the rewards uncertain.

Thomas Kuhn, in *The Structure of Scientific Revolutions*, offers two concepts for thinking about this phenomenon. The first is the concept of the paradigm: once penicillin had clarified the concept of an antibiotic, research on antibiotics proceeded rapidly. What was needed was a clear model of how to proceed. The other is the concept of 'normal' as opposed to 'revolutionary' science. From Hippocrates until the 1870s there was a 'normal' therapeutics, which survived because it was believed to work and, when its efficacy became doubtful, it continued to be employed because patients expected it and doctors could offer nothing better: Louis assumed that a doctor would let the blood of a dying patient, not because there was any prospect of this saving their life, but because it would enable him to assure the family that everything possible had been done. Conventional therapy had enormous stability because both patients and doctors were educated to trust it. That trust carried bloodletting into the twentieth century.

So much, I think, it is easy to see: there were psychological and cultural factors working against innovation. As long as doctors believed they had effective therapies, those factors were sufficient to exclude the microscope from the medical school, and to exclude the theory of animate contagion from practical medicine. From the 1690s to the 1830s the main obstacle to progress in medicine was not some gap in the knowledge, research equipment, or intellectual resources of medical scientists, but rather the psychological and cultural factors which stood in the way of innovations.

The difficult question is whether we need to introduce a further level of argument. After all, precisely when conventional medicine was in a deep crisis, the germ theory came along to rescue it. Was this just luck? Or does it represent some sort of rational adaptation on the part of medical institutions themselves? How you answer this question depends in part on a further question. Do you think institutions have a life of their own? The answer to this question, is, I think, yes. Not being a methodological individualist, I do not think all actions can properly be said to be performed by individuals; some actions are performed by institutions, even though individuals have to be involved as the representatives of the institution. Faced with a range of choices, a committee may reach a decision that was nobody's first choice. In certain circumstances an institution will implement policies that no individual person within the institution thinks are good—this will happen, for example, if an outside agency controls the institution's funding and requires that it meet certain criteria that nobody within the institution actually believes in (a situation not unfamiliar in contemporary universities). This situation was the norm under communism, and is commonplace in institutions that rely on government funding. So there are plenty of circumstances in which an institution can take a decision, or pursue a policy, but there is no simple way in which that decision or policy can be said to be that of any individual within the institution. Institutions can thus take on a life of their own.

So it is legitimate to ask whether there were important institutional constraints obstructing progress in medicine. Did university faculties of medicine, hospitals, or doctors' professional organizations seek to preserve traditional therapies in order to safeguard institutional interests? At the end of Chapter 7 I said that the medical profession turned its back on microscopy: was this the medical profession as a collection of individuals, or as a group of institutions with lives of their own? All the evidence we have seen suggests there was no need for institutions to act; or, where institutions did act, there was no significant gap between those actions and the views of individuals.

Did doctors know what they were doing when they obstructed progress for a century and a half? I've already said that when bad arguments drive out good, those who do the driving must bear the responsibility, but one can be responsible for something one never intended to do—losing one's temper for example. Once doctors decided that they need pay no attention to micro-organisms they immediately ensured that they would never have to encounter evidence suggesting they had made the wrong choice. There are many decisions which have the peculiar characteristic of being self-confirming because you never know what would have happened if you had made a different decision. It is perfectly sensible to say that doctors had no idea what they were doing, but that they bear a burden of responsibility for the consequences of their actions.

After 1830 the microscope came back into fashion, and progress,

effectively halted since the 1680s, recommenced. The new microscopes were much easier to work with than Leeuwenhoek's had been,
and they had the air of being serious scientific instruments. Their
introduction coincided with a crisis in therapy provoked by the
beginning of serious counting. That crisis deepened over the next
few decades. In the 1860s Listerism came to the rescue of the hospitals
when they faced an extremely uncertain future. Without germ
theory the crisis in the hospitals would never have been resolved, and
the hospital as an institution would not have survived.

So the story appears to be one of successful adaptation. Is there any
sense in which we can say that individuals or institutions pursued a
strategy intended to rescue medicine from its crisis? Did the new
knowledge serve institutional purposes? I ask these questions because
the story I have been telling might be of the sort that is labelled
functionalist: according to functionalist arguments, institutions and
social groups react to difficulties by moderating and displacing conflict, allowing their own adaptation and survival. Few people want to
be thought of as functionalists, just as few people want to be thought
of as dyed-in-the-wool Whigs. And yet, just as there ought to be
some histories of progress, so there ought to be some histories that
show how the social order sustains itself, and how it sometimes does
so without any of those who participate in the process fully understanding what they are doing. Functionalist arguments can be
legitimate.

But the account of the revolution in medicine given here is not
intended to be functionalist. Individuals and institutions are naturally
conservative and risk averse. Unless circumstances are very unfavour-
able, they prefer the known to the unknown, continuity to change.
Major change requires a crisis of the sort that hospitals were undergo-
ing in the 1860s: adaptation comes late, not early. Even then change is
likely to be easier to bring about in low-status institutions than in
high-status institutions, on the periphery than in the centre. Listerism
triumphed first in Glasgow, then in Edinburgh; it established itself
quickly in Scotland, but slowly in England. In France, the most
advanced centre of medical research in the early nineteenth century,
germ theory was slower to establish itself among doctors than in

Germany or England. Resistance to innovation is usually most deeply entrenched in those institutions that feel they have most to lose. In such circumstances there is nothing to ensure that institutions will successfully adapt and survive.

It is a remarkable fact that the triumph of germ theory eventually occurred not through a new profession growing up alongside the old profession of medicine, but through doctors adopting the new therapies and (however reluctantly) abandoning the old ones. There was nothing inevitable about this process. Until the discovery of diphtheria serum in 1894, the French medical profession was generally opposed to the new science; then it rapidly converted, and changed the education of doctors to bring it into line with germ theory. Without the discovery of diphtheria serum it is perfectly possible to imagine germ theory continuing to develop in opposition to French medicine, not within it.

From the 1860s on it was clear that germ theory could be applied, whether in silkworm production or surgery. A positive feedback loop was established between research and practice—in the case of medicine between theory and therapy. Once this occurred progress became inevitable and almost irresistible; but it was not inevitable that existing institutions would successfully adapt to this change. Had they failed to do so, there would have been a revolution anyway, even if it had destroyed the existing institutions and fatally weakened the professions of medicine and surgery. Just as there are still homeopaths, so there might still be doctors practising Ionian medicine in Boston and Paris, London and Berlin. Bigger, newer buildings might have sprung up alongside the decaying hospitals of the Ionian doctors, calling themselves Pasteur Institutes or Lister Institutes and dispensing vaccines and antibiotics. It so happens that conventional medicine adapted to germ theory, and it did so because it was very conscious of already being in crisis. But things could easily have turned out differently.

So although germ theory was adopted by the medical profession to serve its purposes, I do not think the story I am telling is functionalist. Germ theory succeeded, not because doctors adopted it, or because it served the purposes of the medical profession, but because it demonstrated a capacity to prolong life, because it was a more effective medical technology than Hippocratic therapy. Germ-theory-based therapy was thus better than Hippocratic therapy at fulfilling the function that conventional medical therapy had claimed to fulfil. This is to take us back to the idea with which the book began, that technologies fulfil functions and establish their own standards of progress. But to agree with that idea is not to commit oneself to 'functionalism' as a doctrine in the social sciences. Rather, it is to accept that there can be standards of rationality that are cross-cultural.

Certain tasks—growing crops, cooking food, postponing death— are common to many cultures. An improved yield, a better irrigation system, a more durable cooking pot, a more effective drug—all these have a logic which is potentially cross-cultural. This does not mean that cross-cultural dissemination is easy or automatic. In the eighteenth century both the French and the English used windmills to grind corn. The English invented the fan-tail, which automatically points the windmill into the wind, and so saves labour. The French never adopted it. Perhaps their labour costs were lower, or their winds less variable, or the capital investment seemed too great. Whatever the reason may be, they certainly understood what the fan-tail was for. So too Lister's contemporaries might have found germ theory puzzling and unconvincing; but they could perfectly understand his claim to have reduced mortality and rendered amputations unnecessary. Arguments for the cultural relativity of rationality have their limits: this is one of the lessons to be drawn from the triumph of germ theory.

IV. AFTER CONTAGION

15
DOLL, BRADFORD HILL, AND LUNG CANCER

I want to end my account of delayed progress in medicine with a final case study. By 1948, when streptomycin was shown to be effective against tuberculosis, it looked as if all the major infectious diseases had been or would soon be conquered. Since then HIV has emerged as a major threat, and other diseases, such as tuberculosis, have developed drug resistance. In our hospitals, death rates from post-operative bacterial infections are rising because of the spread of MRSA (methicillin-resistant staphylococcus aureus), and doctors and nurses, used to relying on antiseptics and antibiotics, are finding it hard to learn new disciplines when it comes to washing hands and changing clothes. A world flu pandemic, we are told, is an imminent possibility. Nevertheless, if we look at the second half of the twentieth century in the developed world then we can think of it as the period after the defeat of the contagious diseases. And as deaths from contagious diseases fell, then of necessity more and more people died from non-contagious diseases: from cancer, heart attacks, strokes. As fast as people suffering from tuberculosis were moved out of hospital wards, people suffering from lung cancer were moved into them.

As doctors turned their attention to these diseases that were far from new, but were suddenly much more important than they had been in the past, they had to abandon the safety of the germ theory of disease which had been the key factor in progress for almost a century. How to make sense of diseases that had no known cause? The first, and still perhaps the greatest, breakthrough was in the study of lung cancer. In 1950 Richard Doll and Austin Bradford Hill published the first major study demonstrating that smoking was the principal cause of lung cancer. I began to take an interest in that article because I read an interview with Richard Doll who said that nobody paid much attention to their research when it was first published; it was only in 1954, when they published a quite different study, or even 1957, when the government agreed that smoking caused lung cancer, that people began to take them seriously. Here, I thought, must be yet another example of bad medicine; as late as 1950 it was evidently still impossible to persuade doctors to take statistical arguments seriously.

The true story, however, is rather different from the story Doll liked to tell in 2004. The interviews with Doll that accompanied the fiftieth anniversary of his 1954 study (and the completion of the research programme announced in that study), and the obituaries that appeared when Doll died the next year consistently misrepresented the true story of the impact of the early work of Doll and Bradford Hill. If I had to summarize that story in a single phrase it would be not 'yet more bad medicine', but 'at last, good medicine'. A consideration of that study provides a fitting end to the main story of this book.

Of the two authors of the 1950 study, Bradford Hill was the senior and the better known. He had published *The Principles of Medical Statistics* in 1937, the first textbook on the subject. It is a mark of the difficulty of teaching doctors statistics at that time that in his book he carefully avoided using the word 'randomization' in the belief that it would scare doctors. But Bradford Hill was, with Philip D'Arcy Hart and Marc Daniels, a member of the team that designed the most famous randomized clinical trial, the one conducted in 1948 on streptomycin as a treatment for tuberculosis. The drug was in such short supply that it had been decided that it was ethical to select by lottery the patients who should be treated with it. Streptomycin was shown to be highly efficacious. ('Efficacious' is here a term of art: drugs are efficacious if they cure patients in trials; they are 'effective' if they cure patients in the real world. Streptomycin turned out to be much less effective than expected because the tubercle bacillus rapidly became resistant to the drug.) The streptomycin trial became a model for all later drug trials.

Bradford Hill and his new colleague Richard Doll (who had

previously carried out a study of the effectiveness of different treatments for ulcers) then turned to an attempt to find out the causes of
lung cancer. Lung cancer rates were rising sharply: in males, the rate
had increased twentyfold between 1905 and 1945. In 1950, the number of deaths from lung cancer, at 13,000, exceeded for the first time
the number of deaths from tuberculosis—which had been falling for
some time. But the cause of the increase in lung cancer was a mystery.
Doll himself suspected that the asphalting of roads might be responsible. Cigarettes were not suspected. Although in Britain legislation in
1908 had banned the sale of cigarettes to children under 16, this was
because cigarettes were thought to stunt growth and so render young
people unfit for military service. There was no generally accepted
view that they were bad for the health of adults, indeed many claimed
that they were good for you.

In order to clear up the mystery as to why lung cancer rates were
on the increase Bradford Hill and Doll (they published as joint
authors) devised a detailed questionnaire to be administered to
patients suspected of having lung cancer—in all 709 patients in London hospitals were interviewed, of whom 649 were men. They were
matched with a control group of 709 hospital patients who were as
like them in every respect as possible, except for the fact that they did
not have lung cancer. In the long list of factors surveyed, one quickly
stood out. Of the male lung cancer patients only 2 were non-smokers;
in the control group 27 were non-smokers. Of the female lung cancer
patients 19 were non-smokers, while in the control group 32 were
non-smokers. A smoker, it should be said, was defined very broadly, as
someone who had smoked at least one cigarette a day for at least a
year in the course of their life. Since we now know smoking causes a
number of diseases, smokers will have been disproportionately present in the control group. A fair guess would be that 80 per cent of
adult men smoked, and 40 per cent of adult women; the men aver-
aging 15 cigarettes a day, and the women half as many. Doll and
Bradford Hill calculated that if there was no statistical connection
between smoking and lung cancer, and thus if the difference between
the two groups was only a matter of chance, then one would have to
conduct the study more than a million times for a difference on this

scale to occur once. These rather small numbers—21 non-smokers amongst the lung cancer patients, 59 in the control group— amounted to proof of a causal connection. Further evidence also showed that the more you smoked the greater the risk: their initial estimate was that heavy smokers were fifty times more likely to die of lung cancer than non-smokers.

One criticism made of this first study was that the results might have been skewed in some way because all the patients in the study came from London. Doll and Bradford Hill quickly conducted a larger survey including patients in Bristol, Cambridge, Newcastle and Leeds, publishing the results in December 1952. These two studies mark the completion of the first phase of their research.

Doll's and Bradford Hill's early work had some distinguished critics, including R. A. Fisher, the first statistician to advocate random trials (Fisher's area of expertise was agriculture rather than medicine, so his were trials of seeds rather than drugs). Fisher pointed out that the fact that there was a statistical correlation did not mean there was a causal link: people with grey hair tend to have short life expectancies, but this is not because grey hair causes death; it is because old age is one of the causes of grey hair, and old age is a major cause of death. There is a real correlation between grey hair and death, but not a causal link. So there might be a genetic trait, for example, which made one both disinclined to smoke and relatively immune to lung cancer. But the crucial fact about Doll's and Bradford Hill's first two publications is that they met with widespread acceptance amongst medical experts. As early as the middle of 1951 the Secretary of the Medical Research Council (which had funded their work) was prepared to state that 'the case against smoking as such is proven' and that there was no need for further statistical work.

Within the new National Health Service, however, there existed a body called the Standing Advisory Committee on Cancer whose job it was to advise on government policy. This committee was reluctant to accept Doll's and Bradford Hill's conclusions, and even more reluctant to see any action based on them. They therefore called in an independent committee of experts, chaired by the government actuary, to reassess the evidence. In November 1953, this committee unequivocally backed Doll and Bradford Hill. As a result, on 12 February 1954, the minister of health, Iain Macleod, announced to the House of Commons that there was a 'real' link (the word 'real' was slightly equivocal—he did not say there was a causal link) between smoking and lung cancer. He went over the same ground at a press conference the same day, smoking as he did so. At that conference the minister tried to walk a tightrope. He had been advised that 'It is desirable that young people should be warned of the risks apparently attendant on excessive smoking', but he insisted that 'the time has not yet come when the Ministry should offer public warnings against smoking'. In other words, the Ministry had accepted that the case against smoking was proven, but they planned to do nothing about it. In this they were following the general policy of the SAC on Cancer, which held that public education about cancer would only provoke anxiety without saving lives.

It is important to stress that the argument that smoking causes cancer had been won by February 1954, because later in life Doll himself used to claim that their research was not taken seriously until later in 1954, with the publication of the first results of an entirely new project, and as a result the 1954 announcement is often presumed to have occurred later in the year, or is confused with an announcement made in 1957. In both 1954 and 1957 the minister announced that smoking was linked to lung cancer, and on both occasions he is supposed to have smoked through the press conference—this story may be true of both occasions, or the two events may have become hopelessly confused.

According to Doll's later account, he and Bradford Hill devised a new statistical study because nobody had taken their early work seriously. The very design of their study shows that this account is wrong. It was funded by a government-appointed body, the Medical Research Council. Its basis was a questionnaire sent in October 1951 to every doctor in the country, all 60,000 of them, by the British Medical Association—it was thus endorsed by the organization that represented all doctors. And finally, it required the active involvement of the Registrar General of Births, Marriages and Deaths, representing another government agency. The second phase of their research was thus only possible because their work had been taken extremely seriously.

Some two-thirds of the doctors approached by Doll and Bradford Hill responded to the questionnaire. The Registrar General then sent Doll and Bradford Hill the death certificate for every doctor who died. By March 1954, 36 doctors who smoked had died of lung cancer, and no non-smoking doctor had done so—since 12.7 per cent of the doctors in their study were non-smokers, nearly 4 should have done so. Their second study thus followed a population over time and showed that smokers died younger than non-smokers. By 1954, Doll and Bradford Hill were already able to point to eleven studies (starting with their own study of 1950) linking smoking and lung cancer. Fifty years later, when the study was finally concluded (the number of doctors alive in 1954 was rapidly diminishing by this point), Doll and Bradford Hill had shown that smoking reduced life expectancy by approximately ten years. They also were able to show by 1956 that stopping smoking, particularly stopping smoking when young, significantly extended life expectancy. Had smoking been banned in 1950, therefore, the whole population (of whom about two-thirds were smokers) would have gained about six years in life expectancy, a gain probably greater than that achieved by the whole of medical science prior to that date. As it is, although lung cancer rates in the UK amongst males peaked in the 1960s as many smokers began to give up, the overall incidence of lung cancer now is still higher than it was in 1950. In 2001 there were 37,500 new cases of lung cancer in the UK.

The accumulation of this new research meant that in 1957 the UK government, although now facing sustained lobbying from the tobacco industry, was finally prepared to accept a 'causal' relationship between smoking and lung cancer—the US Surgeon-General reached the same conclusion at the same time. The UK government's view was based on a report from the Medical Research Council, which had supported Doll's and Bradford Hill's work from the beginning. In fact, it would have been easier to get a straightforward statement on smoking and lung cancer out of the MRC in the autumn of 1952 than it was in 1957: from December 1952 on (partly as a result of the great London smog of 5–12 December 1952 which was thought to have killed 12,000 people) attention increasingly focused on atmospheric pollution as a likely cause of lung cancer, the incidence of which was greater in cities than in the countryside. The *BMJ* editorial which accompanied Doll's and Bradford Hill's publication of 13 December 1952, and which was probably written during the great smog, calculated that air pollution was responsible for roughly 17 per cent of lung cancer deaths, with the rest being attributable to smoking—but it concluded with a call for government action against air pollution, not smoking. The conviction that smog caused disease and death soon led to the Clean Air Act of 1956. In 1957 the MRC initially wanted to issue a statement saying that smoking was the main cause of lung cancer, but that as much as 30 per cent of lung cancer might be caused by atmospheric pollution—a view the government wanted to prevent being articulated, since the government, it was thought, would be held responsible for pollution but not for smoking. At the time no one seems to have made the obvious argument that smokers pollute the air that other people breathe: the key studies showing that passive smoking increases the risk of lung cancer were not made until 1981.

When the MRC's report finally emerged, the *British Medical Journal* at last called for 'the dangers of smoking' to be 'brought home to the public by all the modern devices of publicity'. The government now began, extremely hesitantly, to act: anti-smoking literature was made available, although no real campaign began until the Royal College of Physicians reported in 1962 that smoking caused cancer. By this time, indeed, it was becoming apparent that a range of diseases were associated with smoking. Health warnings were placed on cigarette packets in the US in 1965, but in the UK they were not required until 1971 when experiments on beagle dogs finally showed that you could induce lung cancer by making them breathe cigarette smoke. In the mid-1970s it finally became UK government policy to discourage smoking by raising the tax on cigarettes. By 2000, less than 30 per cent of British men were smokers; the decline in the US had been comparable. Half that decline had taken place by 1970, and thus before the full campaign of health warnings and tax increases had begun.

There are various responses one may reasonably have to this story. One can lament the vast number of lives—worldwide, hundreds of millions of lives—lost because of the failure to ban tobacco, or at least to ban smoking in public places. One can regret that when governments finally acknowledged the nature of the problem, in 1957, the action they took was too little, too late. But you can scarcely argue that the original work undertaken by Doll and Bradford Hill was unreasonably opposed, ignored, or misunderstood. What is impressive is not the small amount of obstruction they faced from the SAC on Cancer (which was opposed to public education on cancers in general), but the speed with which the medical establishment—the BMA, the *BMJ*, the MRC, and those with close links to the medical establishment, such as the government actuary and the Registrar General—acknowledged the importance of their research and sought to foster it. It was this support that made it possible for Doll and Bradford Hill to strengthen their arguments in 1952, 1954, and 1956.

The real puzzles are elsewhere. Late in life, Doll said of their 1950 research, 'When we showed the results to Sir Harold Himsworth, the [Medical Research] Council's Secretary, he said it would have a huge impact. We really thought people would give up immediately.' He himself had given up smoking a few months before—he found it quite easy to do so. Instead the results were completely ignored by the press. On 14 October, a fortnight after Doll's and Bradford Hill's pioneering publication, a letter from D. J. Parr was published in the *British Medical Journal*. It is worth quoting in full:

> Sir, Readers of the popular press are regularly treated to sensational news items based on gleanings from the *Journal* or one of its contemporaries, often before the publication reaches its medical subscribers. In view of the wide range of subjects covered in this way, we must wonder why the usual publicity has not so far been given to the conclusions of Dr. R. Doll and Professor A. Bradford Hill on 'Smoking and Carcinoma of the Lung' (September 30, p. 739)—a topic of much more general interest than the design of perambulators, the dangers of staying in bed, or many others recently in the headlines. Do newspaper editors fear that their public may resent being disillusioned about the 'harmlessness' of the tobacco habit, or are they a little unwilling to risk the displeasure of some of their major advertisers?—I am, etc.

In the very issue in which Doll and Bradford Hill's first research was published, an editorial discussing their work included a wry joke: 'It is said that the reader of an American magazine was so disturbed by an article on the subject of smoking and cancer that he decided to give up reading.' Most journalists were smokers, and far from keen to think about smoking objectively; most of their readers were in the same position. Anti-smoking stories were not likely to sell newspapers to smokers. Another correspondent in 1950, Lennox Johnston, pointed out that smokers could not be trusted to make rational decisions about smoking for the simple reason that they were addicts. He objected to the very language of Doll's and Bradford Hill's paper:

> I take the investigators to task for their 36 references to the habit factor in smoking whilst completely ignoring the much more important craving factor . . . It is . . . a violent euphemism to refer to smoking as a habit. Tobacco smoking is a drug addiction (to be quite precise, a means of administering a drug of addiction, nicotine), and the drug addictions are specific diseases—specific intermittent intoxications . . . Since tobacco smoking is a disease and a preventable one, it is our plain duty to prevent it.

Two years later, when Doll and Bradford Hill published their second paper, another correspondent wrote in to make a similar point. Since a significant proportion of smokers were addicts, there was no point in waiting for people to voluntarily give up smoking. What was needed was a ban on smoking. Had the full significance of these letters been understood, more than twenty years of delay could have been avoided. It was not until the 1980s that the medical profession's attention finally began to focus on the addictive element in smoking.

If there was a major intellectual failure by doctors in 1950, it was not in any failure to understand Doll's and Bradford Hill's research; it was in their failure to recognize that smoking was not a habit but an addiction, and that there was therefore nothing straightforward about persuading people not to smoke. Doll, who suffered from this intellectual failure just as much as everyone else did, never faced it: instead he invented a myth where nobody understood the importance of his and Bradford Hill's work until 1957. But the truth is that by 1950 medicine was becoming powerfully progressive, and new knowledge was eagerly seized upon. Lung cancer proved the first of the non-contagious diseases to be largely preventable, and progress in other fields was much slower. In a hundred years time, historians looking back may identify missed opportunities and unnecessary delays. It's too soon to tell. But the story of this one discovery suggests doctors were quick to appreciate its significance, even if their failure to understand addiction meant that they allowed the government to waste twenty years before taking effective action. Looking back more than fifty years later, Doll thought no one had understood his early work. The truth is they understood it rather well. They just did not know how to act on it.

16
DEATH DEFERRED

In the end we all die: life is a condition with a mortality rate of 100 per cent. Doctors talk of saving lives, but what they really do is defer death. This chapter is about the deaths that medicine has deferred. Deferring death is the main test of medicine's success—not the only one, admittedly, since doctors also alleviate pain and suffering and cure non-fatal conditions. But it is far easier to measure deferred deaths than improved qualities of life. Modern medicine, it turns out, has been far less successful at deferring death than you would think.

The story so far has been straightforward: up until 1865 medicine was almost completely ineffectual where it wasn't positively harmful. Histories of medicine which treat medicine as if it was in some sense 'scientific' and capable of 'progress' before the emergence of a practical germ theory of disease have to keep drawing attention away from this fact, even though it is one that almost no one would deny. After 1865 doctors began to tackle infections with some success. There began to be some real progress in medicine, and this represents the beginning of a new epoch. Recognizing this, it would be easy to conclude that medicine was 'bad' until 1865 (when antiseptic surgery began), or 1885 (when the first modern vaccine was discovered), or 1910 (when salvarsan was introduced as the first effective chemical therapy), or 1936 (when sulphonamides were introduced), or 1942 (when the first antibiotic was introduced), and that thereafter it became, in fairly short order, good medicine, life-saving medicine.

Certainly between 1865 and 1942 doctors began for the first time to defer deaths in significant numbers, but not in numbers anywhere near large enough to explain the astonishing increase in life expectancy that took place during the same period. Medicine has been taking the credit for something that would have happened anyway.

And because there had been a real revolution in life expectancies the impression was created that doctors were rather good at doing what they do. In fact, when it comes to saving lives, doctors have been surprisingly slow and inefficient. For every Semmelweis, horrified at his failure to transform the practice of his contemporaries, there is a Fleming, oblivious in face of a missed opportunity to save lives.

In order to get the achievements of modern medicine in perspective we have to start thinking about life expectancies. What matters is the age at which we die, or (to look at it from another point of view) the proportion of the population that dies each year. If 1 per cent of the population die each year, and if deaths are randomly distributed across ages, then the average life expectancy will be 50. But death does not play fair. It singles out the very young and the very old. In pre-industrial economies something like half those born die by the age of 5; on the other hand a very large proportion of those who survive infancy and early childhood die in their fifties, sixties, and seventies. The result is a life expectancy at birth that rarely rises above 40.

The distribution of deaths across ages in early modern England was such that a death rate of 2.5 per cent per annum corresponded roughly with a life expectancy of 40 years. (The fact that 2.5 goes into a hundred forty times is a coincidence; the relationship between death rate and life expectancy is an empirical one, determined by the distribution of deaths across ages.) The rate first dropped significantly below 2.5 per cent per annum (and life expectancy first rose above 40 years) around 1870, though death rates had intermittently been lower and life expectancies higher in the late sixteenth and early seventeenth centuries.

Medicine has always claimed to be able to postpone death, but there is no evidence that it was able to do so for significant numbers of people before 1942. Between 1900 and 2000, life expectancies in Western countries increased from 45 to 75 years, and death rates fell from 2 to 0.5 per cent. In the course of the last century, death had been deferred by thirty years. This is known as the 'health transition' or the 'vital revolution'. Most people assume that this increase in life expectancy is the result of improvements in medicine, but by 1942 life expectancies had already risen by about twenty years. As a result the extent of medicine's contribution to the health transition is hotly debated. One estimate is that in America modern medicine has increased life expectancy by five years; of those five years, two were gained in the first half of the century, when life expectancy increased by twenty-three years, and three in the second half, when life expectancy increased by seven years. This study implies that Americans owe less than 20 per cent of the increase in life expectancy over the past century to medicine. Another study suggests a figure of 25 per cent for the period 1930 to 1975. A study for the Netherlands proposes that between 4.7 and 18.5 per cent of the increase in life expectancy between 1875 and 1970 was due to direct medical intervention, almost all of it since 1950: in other words, in the region of 12 per cent. The same study estimates that between 1950 and 1980 medical intervention improved the life expectancy of Dutch males by two years and of Dutch females by six years. Thus, according to this research, medical intervention has been the key factor in gains in life expectancy since 1950, but more than three-quarters of the gain in life expectancy took place between 1875 and 1950.

I find these figures hard to believe in the light of my own history: a compound fracture of the arm at the age of 8 would in all probability have killed me before the antiseptic revolution, for I would have been fortunate to survive amputation; and then peritonitis from my burst appendix would certainly have killed me at the age of 13 had I been born anywhere without access to modern surgery: the first appendectomy was performed in 1880. But apparently my own experience is far from typical. The simple fact is that few of us owe our lives to modern medicine.

In order to understand this puzzle we need to explore the changes in health over the last two hundred years. Because evidence is particularly good for England, and because much of the debate over the effectiveness of modern medicine has been concerned with the interpretation of the English evidence, in what follows I am going to concentrate on England, but nothing important would change if we looked at any other modern industrialized country. England is peculiar only in that industrialization and urbanization took place earlier and more rapidly there than anywhere else. Death rates in cities were higher than in the countryside in every Western country until around 1900, so England's exceptionally rapid population growth was achieved despite the braking effect of urbanization. Between 1681 and 1831 the population of England and Wales tripled, from 4.93 million to 13.28 million.

It would seem reasonable to assume that this population increase was largely due to increased life expectancy—that is, to assume that adults are normally sexually active, and that, without birth control, fertility is largely determined by female life expectancy. In the 1680s life expectancy was 32 years; in the 1820s (despite a century of falling wages) it was 39 years, and it was still about the same fifty years later (a fact partly explained by increased urbanization, which shortened lives); it then started a steady climb to 70 in 1960. Thus the first thing to note is that there was a small but significant gain in life expectancy before the first of the modern revolutions in medicine, the victory of germ theory in 1865, took place.

The classic argument that medicine has had almost nothing to do with modern gains in life expectancy is Thomas McKeown's *The Modern Rise of Population* (1976). McKeown's case depended on a series of tables and graphs that showed the proportion of the population killed by a number of key diseases and the way in which this changed over time. Thus respiratory tuberculosis killed 40 people in every 10,000 a year in 1840 and was responsible for 13 per cent of all deaths; this had fallen to 5 deaths in 10,000 by 1945, and yet there was no effective treatment in England until the introduction of streptomycin in 1947. The BCG vaccine had been available from 1921, but its general introduction was delayed because of doubts about its effectiveness—doubts that continue to the present day. Bronchitis, pneumonia and influenza killed 27 in every 10,000 in 1901 (fully 15% of all deaths, for the death rate had fallen by more than 20%); this had halved by the time the first effective treatment, sulphapyridine, was introduced in 1938. Scarlet fever killed 23 in every 10,000 children in 1865; this had fallen to 5 by 1890, and to 1 by the time penicillin, the first effective treatment, was introduced.

Remarkably, then, modern chemical therapies and antibiotics appear on the scene when the major killers have already ceased to kill;

indeed if one looks at the graphs of the death rates, they plunge as fast before the introduction of modern therapies as after. The only possible exception is diphtheria, which killed 9 in every 10,000 children in 1895 when antitoxins were first used in treatment, and the death rate from which had fallen to 3 by 1920, though the role of antitoxins in this decline is a matter of dispute, as a similar decline took place in America before the introduction of antitoxins. Of the major fatal diseases in 1850, only bronchitis, pneumonia and influenza were still killing significant numbers in 1970: 5 in every 10,000, or 11 per cent of all deaths.

Disease after disease appears to have lost much of its capacity to kill long before there was anything resembling an effective treatment. In one case, scarlet fever, the disease itself seems to have declined in virulence. In every other case, either the external environment had become less favourable to the micro-organisms responsible, or human beings had become better at resisting infection. In 1850, 60 per cent of all deaths were caused by micro-organisms; in 1900 it was 50 per cent; in 1970 it was under 15 per cent. (People were now dying of heart disease and cancer rather than pneumonia and tuberculosis.) The germs had been very largely defeated, but the new drugs played only a small part in this triumph.

The same picture appears if we turn from disease to childbirth. In England death in childbirth was around 160 mothers in every 10,000 births in 1650; this had fallen to 55 by 1850, a level that continued almost unaltered at least until the introduction of prontosil in 1935. Thereafter the level falls sharply to close to 1 in 10,000 in the 1980s. This is not how it ought to be. Once Lister had formulated antiseptic principles, deaths in childbirth should have fallen sharply, and indeed did in countries that relied on well-educated midwives. In England however, busy general practitioners refused to take adequate antiseptic precautions and death rates remained far higher than they should have been. The shape of the curve for deaths in childbirth is very different from that for deaths from infectious diseases, but again there are major gains before 1865, even if the impact of modern medicine was significant and immediate after 1935. Here the major advance prior to antibiotics was the introduction of the obstetrical forceps, at first a secret in the Chamberlen family, but in widespread use after 1730.

Apart from obstetrical forceps, were there any other successful interventions to extend life expectancy before the 1860s? One case that calls for consideration is the disappearance of bubonic plague from Western Europe. Bubonic plague killed large numbers of people between its first European occurrence in 1348 and the mid-seventeenth century. In the 1650s it ceased to attack Italy, in the 1660s England became plague free, and France suffered only a small and final outbreak in Marseilles in the 1720s. Some hold that this fearsome disease (which killed 225,000 people in London between 1570 and 1670) was conquered by quarantine measures, but this claim is impossible to prove. Plague is carried by rat fleas, and is primarily a disease of rats that happens also to infect humans. If its primary means of spreading was from rat to flea to rat, then quarantining humans could only have had a limited effect on the movement of rats and fleas. Early modern doctors believed quarantine would work because they thought the disease was quite exceptional in that it could (at least in epidemic circumstances) be spread directly from human to human, even though they believed it was originally caused by a corruption of the air. Although working with a false theory, they certainly had some success in protecting individual cities from plague some of the time; but whether their measures were capable of eradicating the disease from Western Europe as a whole, or (if it was never endemic) of preventing its periodic reintroduction, is more doubtful. Probably an alternative explanation in terms either of the declining virulence of the disease or of changes in the rat population (plague infects black rats, not brown) is to be preferred. With the possible exception of bubonic plague, there is only one major success story prior to 1865 that needs to be considered: smallpox.

The first demonstrably effective intervention against micro-organisms was vaccination, which offered an effective method of prevention. Jenner introduced vaccination against smallpox in 1796. The effects were extraordinary: there were 12,000 deaths from smallpox in Sweden in 1800 (approximately 15 per cent of all deaths), and just 11 in 1822, although only 40 per cent of the susceptible population had been vaccinated. Vaccination made possible the final elimination of smallpox throughout the globe in 1978. In England, vaccination was preceded by inoculation with live virus, which became fairly widespread from the 1750s. On the other hand, uptake of both inoculation and vaccination was sporadic and patchy compared to those countries such as Sweden and Prussia that made systematic use of Jenner's vaccine. In the 1680s in London at least 7 per cent of all deaths were attributable to smallpox, and by 1850 this had fallen to 1 per cent. The figure of 7 per cent is almost certainly an underestimate. In London the cause of death was recorded by laypeople; elsewhere, where it was recorded by doctors, smallpox seems to have been responsible for 14 per cent of deaths.

This implies that inoculation and vaccination were responsible for something like half the increase in life expectancy in England during the period 1680 to 1850. Let us take Bernoulli's unduly conservative estimate, that inoculation increased life expectancy by two years, and compare this with the average gain in life expectancy attributable to modern medicine of four years in Holland between 1950 and 1980. If one thinks of the vast investment in research laboratories, hospitals, drug companies, and general practitioners dedicated to increasing life expectancy in the period between 1950 and 1980, it is striking that the result was at best only equivalent to the conquest of smallpox twice over. Fifty years after Jenner's discovery, John Snow called it both 'the greatest discovery that has ever been made in the practice of medicine' and 'the greatest benefit' that humankind 'have probably ever received'. It comes as something of a shock to realize that this may still be true.

Modern vaccination therapies in human beings (based on the identification of the infective agent, which Jenner was unable to make) begin with Pasteur's vaccination against rabies in 1885. But, apart from diphtheria, there was no major breakthrough against a disease that killed significant numbers in the West prior to the BCG vaccine against tuberculosis (and even the BCG is questionable). The major impact of vaccinations (against polio in 1957, for example, or rubella in 1963) came after, not before the first antibiotics, and falls in the period 1950–80.

So what did cause the long-term doubling of life expectancy in England from 32 in 1680 to 65 in 1942? There is general agreement that medicine was not responsible and that McKeown is therefore right in his central claim, but it is much harder to work out what exactly was responsible. We are in the profoundly unsatisfactory situation of not having anything resembling an adequate understanding of the most important single event in modern history, the revolution in life expectancy. McKeown thought he knew the answer. He argued that the major factor was better resistance to disease, and that the only thing that could have made this possible was better nutrition. His argument has come under repeated and sustained attack, but it remains the best explanation we have.

On some things McKeown was certainly wrong. He was certainly wrong to think that, until contraception, fertility varies less than mortality. We now know that, although there is a modest increase in life expectancy between 1680 and 1820, two-thirds of the English population increase over that period was caused by increased fertility—and birth rates continued to rise until 1870. Part of this increased fertility resulted from a higher rate of marriage (the proportion of women never marrying dropped from 15 per cent to half of that); part from earlier marriage (the average age for first marriage fell by three years); and part from increased procreation outside marriage (in 1680 less than one tenth of all first births were illegitimate, while in 1820, 25 per cent were).

Earlier marriage and a higher proportion marrying could in principle be the result of rising standards of living, which would make it easier for people to afford to start a family, but in fact the fit between rising fertility and rising standards of living is not very good. It seems clear that in the early modern period fertility was kept in check by deliberate abstinence on the part of the unmarried, and that in the course of the eighteenth and nineteenth centuries abstinence became much less popular. In short, people became more sexually active. There is no adequate study of why this might be, but a reasonable guess is that it reflects the decline in the church courts and of other mechanisms, formal and informal, of policing sexual behaviour. The history of population increase before 1870, in England at least, turns out to have more to do with the history of sexual activity (including sex within marriage) than with the history of life expectancy. Smallpox inoculation and vaccination may have been responsible for one-third of the increase in life expectancy, but they can only explain one-ninth of the increase in population. The primary cause of population increase, at least in England, was an increase in sexual activity, a possibility which McKeown never suspected although his subject was 'the modern rise in population'.

Second, McKeown chose to concentrate his attention not just on diseases caused by germs, but on diseases caused by airborne germs. Of the increase in life expectancy between 1850 and 1970, 40 per cent was due to the declining death rate from these diseases—tuberculosis, bronchitis, pneumonia, influenza, whooping cough, measles, diphtheria, and smallpox. The most important single cause of improved life expectancy was the decline in the death rate from tuberculosis. The consequence of McKeown's concentration on airborne diseases was that standard public health measures, which had conventionally been assumed to be a major factor in rising life expectancy, suddenly seemed irrelevant. Piped water, sewers, and water-closets are completely irrelevant to the spread of TB.

What then were the obstacles to the spread of TB? Once the bacillus had been identified by Koch in 1882 people knew that they were dealing with an airborne germ, and public health campaigns against spitting might well have had some impact on the spread of infection. When I was a child there were still signs on buses in England (and in France) telling passengers not to spit. Perhaps the isolation of sufferers in sanatoria might also have served to protect the uninfected population. Yet arguments like these break down in face of a simple fact: 85 per cent of young people in 1946 had antibodies that showed they had been exposed to TB. Thus the TB germ was still clearly widespread. What seems to have changed is not the proportion of the population being exposed to TB, but the proportion dying as a result of exposure.

In fact this seems to be true of disease in general. Three surveys of a friendly society, delightfully named the Odd Fellows, enable us to assess the incidence of sickness in the working-class population in

1847, 1868, and 1895. What we discover is that there was no decline in the rate at which people fell ill. What declined was the proportion of illnesses that resulted in death. McKeown is right: the germs were still there, but the people were better able to survive them.

Third, McKeown's preoccupation with airborne diseases meant that he paid little attention to the history of sanitation. In the period 1850 to 1900, the reduction of death from water- and food-borne diseases was almost as important as the reduction in death from airborne diseases. London began to introduce sand filtration of the water supply in 1828. Chemical treatment of sewage water was common in the 1860s—it was in part this that gave Lister the idea of antiseptic surgery. The construction of a modern sewage-treatment system in London began in 1858. Generally across England, investment in improvements to water and sewage was highest in the last two decades of the century. Public health measures were clearly crucial in eliminating cholera, which between appearing in England for the first time in 1831 and for the last in 1866, caused in all some 113,000 deaths. The conquest of cholera has always been an exciting chapter in the history of medicine, but this success needs to be kept in proportion. Cholera itself was responsible for barely more than 0.5 per cent of all deaths, whereas whooping cough, for example, was responsible for 1.5 per cent, or 300,000 deaths in the cholera years.

It is particularly striking that while adult deaths from diarrhoea and dysentery fell sharply during the period of public health investment (in the 1890s the overall rate was three-quarters of what it had been forty years earlier, and amongst young adults it was one-tenth of what it had been then), death rates among children actually rose. At the beginning of the twentieth century roughly 3 per cent of English children under the age of 5 died from diarrhoea and dysentery, but the death toll rose to 5 per cent in years when there was a hot summer. By the 1930s, however, the death rate for children was one-tenth what it had been thirty years earlier: some important change had taken place in the intervening period.

Evidently piped water and treated sewage, which were widespread by the end of the nineteenth century, did not significantly reduce children's exposure to water- and food-borne micro-organisms.

Adults seem to have been less exposed than before—even among the very elderly, whom one would expect to be highly susceptible, death rates were one third what they had been. However they also seem to have become more resistant, hence the steeper decline amongst young adults than the elderly. By contrast, nothing at all happened until the 1910s and 1920s to reduce the exposure of small children. How can we make sense of this rather bizarre pattern? Adults became more resistant to waterborne disease, but were also less exposed to it; while infants and small children were as vulnerable as before.

A 1910 study found that diarrhoea (which mainly occurred amongst children) was as common in households that had flush toilets as in those that did not. Modern sanitation was thus quite ineffectual. Why? Because young children still went to the toilet in the street and played amongst faeces. Children were thus far more susceptible to diarrhoea than adults, and adults must then have been primarily exposed to germs through their contact with children. From the 1890s on it became increasingly common for health visitors to pay regular visits to families after the birth of a child (a practice which became virtually universal after the 1907 Notification of Birth Acts), bringing with them theories of disease transmission which were far from new, but which had previously not been properly disseminated amongst the working classes.

It has been argued that it was only in the twentieth century that 'domestic micro-sanitation came to supplement urban macro-sanitation, resulting in improvements more dramatic than any of those achieved in the nineteenth century'. By 'domestic micro-sanitation' is meant not only cleaning and scrubbing, but using nappies, and potty training; washing hands after going to the bathroom; and the killing of flies and the covering of food. It is striking that where the average age for potty training is now twenty-four months an expert in 1839 thought that nappies could be abandoned at four months—a strategy which implies a universal acceptance of frequent 'accidents'.

Hygiene had been improving for centuries. In the sixteenth century people ate off slabs of bread ('trenchers'), in the seventeenth off wooden plates, in the eighteenth off pewter, and in the nineteenth off ceramic. Most people in the nineteenth century seem to have washed their hands and their faces every day. In the seventeenth century heavy woollen clothing (made of broadcloth) was replaced by lighter new draperies, and in the eighteenth and nineteenth centuries wool was replaced by cotton. As a result clothes could be washed much more easily and the consumption of soap rose from 3.5 pounds per person per year in 1800 to 8 pounds in 1861 (more soap was surely used washing clothes than washing bodies). Already in 1801 William Heberden thought he could show an astonishing reduction in deaths from diarrhoea through the course of the eighteenth century as a result of increased cleanliness and better ventilation.

In the late nineteenth century public bath houses were built for the urban working classes: in 1852 Parisians took on average 3.7 public baths each a year; there is no way of counting the baths they may have taken at home. When the Pasteur Institute was built in 1888 it stood close to the factory manufacturing Eau de Javel or domestic bleach—the case for cleanliness was clear long before the triumph of the germ theory of disease. By the beginning of the twentieth century most new English houses had running water, flush toilets and baths, but what is clear from the English evidence is that much of this improvement in hygiene had little effect on life expectancies. Children in particular continued to die in the same numbers as before.

What had happened was that Heberden had misunderstood his own statistics: deaths from 'griping in the guts' had just been reclassified by doctors as deaths from 'convulsions'. It took a systematic application of the principles of the sanitary reformers to domestic life to conquer infantile diarrhoea; there was no need to wait for germ theory. What needed to be done had been clear since (at least) Edwin Chadwick's *Report on the Sanitary Condition of the Labouring Population of Great Britain* (1842), but it took almost a hundred years to transform childrearing practices.

If we look for deliberate interventions to reduce disease prior to the 1930s there are some important examples: quarantine against plague, obstetric forceps, vaccination against smallpox, macro- and micro-sanitation. Forceps deliveries and smallpox vaccinations were mainly administered by doctors, and quarantine and sanitation drew extensively on medical theories. But none of these developments can account for the extraordinary increase in life expectancies from the 1870s onwards. Here we have to return to McKeown's contentious claim that the explanation lies with improved nutrition.

At first it seems as though McKeown must be wrong on this crucial question. We now know that England was the first country in Europe to escape periods of high mortality caused by bad harvests. From the early seventeenth century there was enough food, not only enough to prevent people from starving, but enough to prevent people from being so weakened by malnutrition that they succumbed in significant numbers to infections in years of bad harvests and high food prices. If malnutrition caused, as McKeown argues, high death rates, then surely death rates should be higher in these years? Since there is virtually no increase of this sort, McKeown would appear to be wrong.

Or perhaps not. Adults in England in 1775, as we now know, were 10 cm or 4 inches shorter than they are at present—similar or larger differences are to be found in all Western countries with the exception of America, where the gap (amongst the white population) is smaller. Modern data demonstrate a remarkable correlation between height and life expectancy. Research in Norway shows that a middle-aged man who is 5ft 5 in. is 70 per cent more likely to die over a sixteen-year period than a man of the same age who is 6ft tall. A person's final height crucially depends on two things, apart from their genetic inheritance: nutrition in infancy and in childhood, and exposure to disease while growing. Robert Fogel has argued that, if one compares heights in the US (where meat was already plentiful in the mid-nineteenth century), England, and other Western European countries, one can form the impression that 60 per cent of the difference between modern English heights and those in 1775 is due to improved nutrition, and 40 per cent to reduction in exposure to disease (which is mainly a twentieth-century phenomenon). Moreover, improved nutrition in infancy and childhood, as reflected in increased height, explains almost all the increase in life expectancy before 1875 and 50–75 per cent of the increase after 1875 (when public health measures and modern medicine begin to play a significant role).

McKeown's thesis that increased life expectancy is due to improved nutrition is thus, if one accepts Fogel's argument, broadly correct, but it requires one simple modification: what is crucial is nutrition in infancy and childhood, and here what matters is not just the number of calories consumed, but also the consumption of protein and vitamins. Meat consumption was far higher in the US than in Europe: in France in 1870 it was about 40 per cent of what it was in the US at the same date, and as a consequence Americans were on average some 5 cm taller than the French, and significantly longer lived. If Fogel is correct, the fact that the English were rarely so malnourished as to die within weeks or months of a bad harvest is irrelevant; through into the twentieth century they (and particularly the poorest amongst them) were generally sufficiently malnourished during infancy and childhood for their long-term life expectancy to be adversely affected. More recent work suggests that nutrition in the womb may be even more important than nutrition in infancy. Thus at the moment the best explanation for increases in life expectancy between the 1870s and the 1930s is improvement in foetal and childhood nutrition, and improved nutrition continues to be a major factor (though perhaps no longer the major factor) in rising life expectancy down to the present day.

How much has modern medicine contributed to the increase in life expectancy? The answer seems to be about 20 per cent, much less than improved nutrition and improved sanitation. From 1865 onwards, doctors have become increasingly good at deferring death, but surprisingly few of us owe our lives to modern medicine. It is easy to adopt a patronizing attitude to those patients who, from 425 BC to 1865, imagined their doctors were doing them good when they were only doing them harm. But we too are credulous. We owe much less to modern medicine than we imagine.

CONCLUSION

Primum non nocere.
First do no harm.
(Thomas Inman, 1860)

Three simple arguments run through this book. The first is that if we define medicine as the ability to cure diseases, then there was very little medicine before 1865. The long tradition that descended from Hippocrates, symbolized by a reliance on bloodletting, purges, and emetics, was almost totally ineffectual, indeed positively deleterious, except in so far as it mobilized the placebo effect.

The second is that effective medicine could only begin when doctors began to count and to compare. They had to count the number of patients that lived and the number that died, and then compare different treatments to see if they resulted in improved survival rates. The idea of counting and comparing seems a very simple one, and yet doctors were very slow to put it into practice. This is partly because counting and comparing is in fact a rather complex cultural activity, much facilitated by the introduction of devices such as the table for organizing information. It is also because before you can count and compare you need to have a conception of disease that makes counting and comparing possible. By the beginning of the nineteenth century counting and comparing was inescapable, and within fifty years medicine was in crisis because it was clear that conventional therapies did not work.

Thirdly, the key development that made modern medicine possible is the germ theory of disease. More specifically, the first breakthrough took place with the germ theory of putrefaction. The great puzzle here is the long delay before anyone formulated a germ theory that had a medical application. As early as 1597, Felix Platter had formulated a sophisticated germ theory of contagion. In 1677 Leeuwenhoek had seen germs through his microscope. A series of scientists, including Leeuwenhoek himself, had denied that germs were spontaneously generated. By 1714, if not earlier, the old seeds of disease theories had been fully adapted in the light of Leeuwenhoek's discoveries. In 1752 Pringle was working on antiseptics. As early as 1810 it was evident that there was something seriously wrong with existing theories of putrefaction. Yet the first disease caused by a germ (in silkworms) was not identified until 1835; the germ theory of putrefaction was not formulated until 1837; and the first application of germ theory to medicine did not occur until 1865. How to explain this delay? Some have attributed it in large part to the inadequacy of early microscopes, but the evidence suggests they are wrong. It is true that there were conceptual obstacles to be overcome, but it is difficult to see that those obstacles were major ones. All the evidence suggests that the delay in formulating a practical germ theory has its origin not within microbiology but outside it. The chief obstacle was that doctors were satisfied with their existing therapies; the barriers to progress were psychological and cultural not intellectual.

In pursuing these arguments I have deliberately broken one written and a number of unwritten rules. I have focused on progress, which historians are not supposed to do. That rule is written in places where all historians have read it. The unwritten rules are harder to identify, but here are two. First, a history book should have a homogeneous character, so that one can easily say this book is about therapy, or this book is about the origins of the germ theory of disease. I have quite deliberately not written a book like that.

My model has, let me confess, been Fernand Braudel's great work, *The Mediterranean in the Age of Philip II* (1949), written in a prisoner-of-war camp, without access to books or notes. His book is really three books in one. The first deals with continuity, with things that changed hardly at all between the ancient Romans and the eighteenth century: trade routes, the distribution of crops, the technology of transport. The second deals with things that changed over the course of decades: inflation, banditry, styles of architecture. And the third deals with a political crisis and a military campaign, with events that changed from day to day.

This book, while less ambitious, still amounts to three books in one. In the first part, I have surveyed a tradition of therapy that survived from Hippocrates until the early twentieth century. In the second part and the beginnings of the third I have given an account of a world which begins with Vesalius and ends with Claude Bernard, a world in which medical knowledge progressed, but in which that knowledge had little or no significance for therapy. Then in the rest of the third part I have described, in very brief outline, the emergence of a world in which medical knowledge established a positive feedback loop with medical therapy: progress in knowledge led to progress in therapy, which led to more investment in research. That is the world in which we still live, and in the last chapter I discussed how much we have gained as a result of medical progress.

And that brings me to the second unwritten rule that I have broken. History books on big subjects are supposed to be 'big' books. This is not a big book, in that sense, but a book which makes an argument. What counts is getting the basic framework right. If that framework is correct, then it becomes evident where we may need a longer and more detailed story of what actually happened: we may need to know more, for example, about theories of animate contagion before Pasteur (a field in which research effectively stopped twenty years ago), more about the renaissance of microscopy in the 1830s, more about the crisis in medical therapy between the 1830s and the 1890s. In this way Braudel's *Mediterranean* amounted to a programme for research, and it doubled in size between its first publication in 1949 and the revised 2nd edition in 1966. Perhaps this book too has the potential for future growth.

So what kind of argument have I developed here? In 1962, Thomas Kuhn published *The Structure of Scientific Revolutions*. In that book he introduced a number of key concepts. He distinguished sharply between 'normal science' and the science that takes place during periods of crisis. His argument was that major intellectual advances only take place in the context of a crisis within existing ways of thinking and doing: my argument is that something that we may call 'normal medicine' was carried on from Hippocrates until the 1850s. Intellectual and practical problems were solved, new ideas such as the circulation of the blood were incorporated, but the foundational assumption, the Hippocratic method of therapy, went largely unquestioned (despite the efforts of Paracelsus and van Helmont). Real progress began only when that assumption began to be questioned.

Kuhn also argued that what held science together were what he called 'paradigms'. He used the word in a number of different senses. A paradigm might be a laboratory activity, learnt by generations of students, such as cultivating a pure sample of a bacterium in a petri dish. It might be a model solution to a problem, such as Pasteur's development of a vaccine against anthrax, a model that could then be adapted and applied to other diseases. It might be the epitome of something you needed to know to belong to an intellectual community: you could not hope to understand the publications of the Institut Pasteur without some knowledge of Pasteur's work on anthrax and rabies, and of the work his followers had done on diphtheria, because that provided the common stock of references that others relied on in explaining their own work. Thus one could give an account of a paradigm that related it to a practice, a theory, or a sociological community. As a consequence Kuhn's account of science was radically unstable—one could conclude from it that in order to understand science one needed to look closely at what scientists actually did in laboratories; or to study closely the way in which textbooks evolved over time; or to look at the structure of authority that held a community together—at what happened, for example, when an outsider submitted a paper to the Institut Pasteur to be published.

The argument I have presented here represents one choice amongst these three options, each of which can claim to have been endorsed by Kuhn. The primary obstacle to progress, as I have argued, was not practical (Leeuwenhoek's microscopes worked well), nor theoretical (the germ theory of putrefaction was not difficult to formulate), but psychological and cultural. It lay in doctors' sense of themselves, their awareness of their own traditions, their habit of conferring authority upon an established canon and upon established therapies. Doctors successfully pushed the microscope, and all the questions that it generated, out of medicine in the 1690s, and kept it

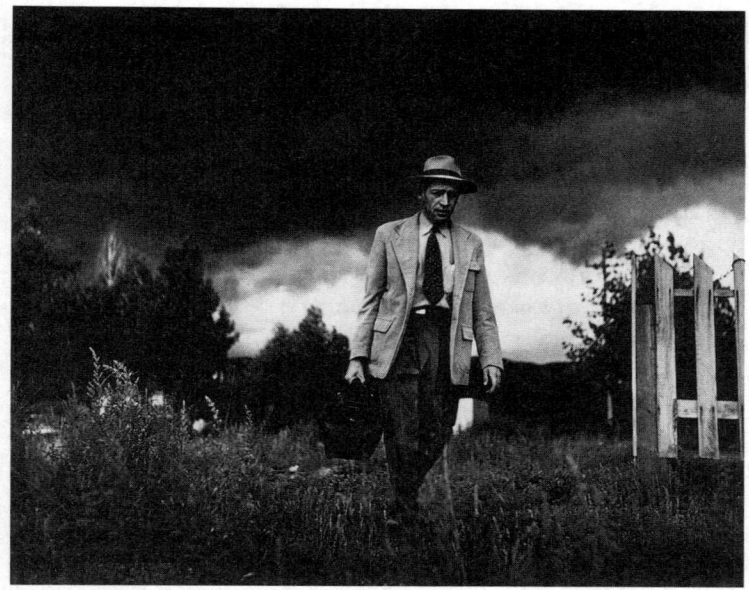

32. W. Eugene Smith, *Dr Ceriani Making a House Call*, 1948. From a photographic essay entitled 'The Country Doctor' published in *Life*.

out until the 1830s. They did so because they saw it as a threat to traditional medicine, and they dealt with that threat so successfully that they extended the life of traditional medicine by a century and a half.

Medicine is an activity that is deeply embedded in institutions and in social practices, and that makes heavy demands on the psyche. For other forms of knowledge, a quite different type of account may be necessary. In physics, the key barriers to progress may be theoretical. In oceanography they may be practical. So too, in other periods of medicine a different type of account may be necessary. It is too soon to tell, for example, what the obstacles to making progress in curing cancer have been; they may prove to be quite different in character to the obstacles encountered by germ theory.

I have chosen to place my argument in the context of Kuhn

because history of medicine, as I understand it, is largely post-Foucauldian when it ought to be post-Kuhnian. Under the influence of a historical profession opposed to the discussion of progress on the one hand and a postmodernist intellectual tradition committed to relativism on the other, historians of medicine have been unable to think about the different types of progress that can occur in medicine, and have failed to ask what keeps the crucial paradigms shared by doctors in place.

Let me turn my own method of argument against myself. Why was the book that I have just written not written thirty or forty years ago? There was perhaps a window of opportunity, between 1962 and 1976, and it would be interesting to go back and review the histories of medicine written in those years to see if any of them are similar to this. But that window was only ajar: it was still easy, in those years, to think that Leeuwenhoek's microscopes were inferior to those of the 1830s. And it was soon closed. Under the triple impact of Foucault, of Illich, and of McKeown, the very idea of progress in medicine came to seem a naïve and simplistic one. Of those three authors, Illich and McKeown no longer have the influence they once had; only Foucault remains as a major obstacle. The idea of progress now needs to be rescued from the condescension of Butterfield and of Foucault.

POSTSCRIPT, 2007

'great truths may be very near and yet not be discerned'

Sir James Paget, 1879

Opinion about *Bad Medicine* is polarized. Broadly speaking, doctors (who take progress seriously) love it, and historians of medicine and of science (who don't) hate it. Since the book is about the way in which a profession can become wedded to irrational and unjustifiable assumptions, and since it calls in question mainstream medical history, it would be disconcerting if the historians had greeted it with enthusiasm. In fact the reception of *Bad Medicine* has been a striking example of just the kind of resistance to innovation that the book itself analyses.

One reason *Bad Medicine* has polarized opinion is that its own argument is conducted in terms of polarities: good medicine and bad medicine, heroes and villains. The question of whether it is permissible to write 'accusatory' or 'celebratory' history is the most interesting one raised by the critics, and it is evident that I did not address it fully in the book's opening pages. There are in fact a number of interlocking issues that need to be prised apart. First, my opponents advocate what anthropologists call 'charitable interpretation': we should understand the past in its own terms, and make our best efforts to bring out the rationality of viewpoints which at first seem alien to us. The problem with charitable interpretation as a methodological principle is that it is designed for societies in which everyone thinks more or less alike. But if you want to understand a dispute (and there have been disputes about medicine since the days of Hippocrates) understanding one side's point of view 'in its own terms' involves criticizing the other side; a 'charitable interpretation' of one side's arguments is of necessity a 'stranger's account' of the other side's. There is no choice: as I say, 'You have to take sides.' For a striking example of this see Steven Shapin's and Simon Schaffer's *Leviathan and the Air Pump* (1986), in which they take Thomas Hobbes's side against Robert Boyle on the question of the possibility of a vacuum.

A crucial difference between *Leviathan and the Air Pump* and *Bad Medicine* is that Shapin and Schaffer defend what looks to us like the losing side, while I give my support to those scientists and doctors who turned out, as we see it, to be in the right. It is not taking sides that my critics really object to, I think; it is taking *this* side. History is written for the living, not the dead, so every history book, whether avowedly or only implicitly, is an intervention in our own culture and involves some sort of taking of sides: historians of science who refuse to write about progress are, explicitly or implicitly, questioning the role of science in our own society. What is shocking about *Bad Medicine* is that it quite openly employs hindsight to decide which side to take. Critics who say that it relies on 'twenty-twenty hindsight' or on the use of what doctors call a 'retrospectoscope' are making a serious point. There's no doubt, for example, that the book looks closely at early germ theories of disease because the germ theory of disease turned out to be broadly correct, and this is a judgment made with the benefit of hindsight. There are plenty of theories—those of Paracelsus, or van Helmont, for example—that *Bad Medicine* passes over quickly, because with hindsight we know they were incorrect.

Argument from hindsight is not always bad history, and I want first to present two reasons for thinking such arguments are permissible, and then later I will go even further and claim that in history of science hindsight is indispensable. Let us think, for a moment, not about curing diseases, but about propulsion. For people in the seventeenth century there were only three reliable forces of propulsion: human and animal muscle power (horses, oars, etc.); the wind (sails on boats and on windmills); and water (watermills). Within these three broad categories of power-source there were all sorts of improvements that were possible—the introduction of the fan-tail on windmills for example (1745), or the invention of the bicycle. It makes sense to ask what the preconditions for those improvements were: Why was the fan-tail never adopted in France? Why was the bicycle not invented until 1865? And there was of course a power source that everybody had some experience of, but whose significance had simply not been recognized: steam. Thomas Savery patented the first steam engine in 1698, although Hero of Alexander had already used steam power in the first century AD, as had Giambattista della Porta in 1606.

In a pre-electrical world there is a finite, and specifiable, set of possible sources of power. One can call it *hindsight* that enables us to identify them as muscle power, wind power, water power, and steam power, but one can also call it *insight*. Some lines of enquiry were promising, others (perpetual motion machines, for example) were doomed to failure. We can say this because there are objective limits on which technologies will work and which ones will not, and it is therefore interesting and productive to ask what the obstacles were to inventing the steam engine before 1698, the fan-tail before 1745, or the bicycle before 1865. A history of technology which treated perpetual motion machines in the same way as it treated steam engines would be strange indeed. However some people insist that this is exactly how history of science should proceed. They advocate what is called the 'symmetry principle'—that one should give the same kind of account of false beliefs as of true beliefs, of irrational beliefs as of rational beliefs. *Bad Medicine* does not respect the symmetry principle, and it would be irrational to do so.

Others, who do not go quite as far as to adopt the symmetry principle, still do not think that science is constrained by objective limits. If you think science is socially constructed, then the number of possible sciences is infinite, and the sciences you actually get are a purely contingent and unpredictable outcome. If you think like this, then hindsight always misses the point, which is that the future could not possibly have been predicted. This seems to me plain wrong about science, and particularly about technology. Technologies develop in directions that are constrained by the laws of nature, and by and large (with the interesting exceptions of astrology, alchemy, and Hippocratic medicine) fantasy technologies are easy to identify and are quickly abandoned. There were no *alternatives* to the steam engine in the sense that there might be alternatives to constitutional monarchy, or utilitarianism, or tragic drama, or the morse code. Once a serious search for a new power source began, it was only a matter of time before the steam engine was invented. So too, if medicine was to become effective, there was no *alternative* to the germ theory of disease, or to its application in the form of vaccines, antiseptics, and antibiotics. One can imagine a different timing and pace of progress (indeed I argue we need to take seriously the idea that the timing and pace of progress could have been very different); one cannot conceive of progress taking place in a quite different direction. In situations like this it is perfectly permissible to use hindsight in order to concentrate one's attention on valid lines of enquiry, to ask what the obstacles to them were and how they were overcome. This does not mean that one should ignore failed lines of enquiry (the history of perpetual motion machines is of real interest): but there is no need to treat them as if they could have succeeded.

There is a second version of the argument about hindsight that also looks, at first, as if it deserves to be taken seriously. In this book I frankly admit that if we are going to talk about 'good' medicine (medicine which works) and 'bad' medicine (medicine which performs worse than a placebo, and may do harm), then we are also going to have to praise and blame individuals who were able to tell one from the other. My critics take exception to this way of thinking, and yet I am grateful to one of them, Chris McManus, for an example that shows that it comes naturally to people caught up in the midst of an intellectual revolution. He reports that Sir James Paget, the Victorian surgeon and pathologist, looking back in 1879, was dismayed and puzzled when he realized how unnecessary had been the delay in inventing anaesthetic surgery, reflecting how 'great truths may be very near and yet not be discerned.' 'In explanation,' McManus says,

> Paget emphasizes 'the misery (of painful operations) was so frequent, so nearly customary, deemed so inevitable that, though it excited horror... it did not excite to strenuous action'... Paget did not expect a kindly verdict from history: 'Our successors... will look back with horror, and on us with wonder and contempt for what they will call our idleness or blindness or indifference to suffering.'

What could be wrong with writing precisely the sort of history that Paget foresaw, a history that looks back with horror and wonder at idleness, or blindness, or indifference to suffering?

In 1930, Cecil Paine, working in Sheffield, was the first doctor (or at least the first since Lister) to make clinical use of penicillin. Paine, who had read Fleming's 1929 article on penicillin, used 'crude mould juice' to treat eye infections that were resistant to all available therapies—gonorrheal infections in the eyes of newborn babies, and a pneumococcus infection in the eye of a man injured in an industrial accident. He had remarkable success, but abandoned his work when he was posted to a new job. Wainwright and Swan, who have written the history of Paine's work with penicillin, defend his failure to recognize the potential of mould juice. We must, they say, avoid hindsight, and recognize that in the 1930s doctors were looking for antiseptics not antibiotics. But Paine himself took a different view. 'At the end of our interview Dr Paine was asked where he placed himself in the penicillin story. He replied: "Nowhere—a poor fool who didn't see the obvious when it was stuck in front of him".' Both Wainwright and Swan on the one hand, and Paine on the other are right: it would have been remarkable if Paine had grasped the full implications of the cures he was performing; but it is also true to say that the obvious was stuck in front of him—and he, after all, was alone at the time in having grasped the significance of Fleming's 1929 article, alone in having started to use penicillin to kill off infections, so that the obvious was stuck in front of someone who really *was* more than half way to grasping its significance. Contempt seems entirely the wrong response here, but a certain amount of wonder and dismay is surely in order. Since participants in the events see no problem in employing hindsight, historians too should be allowed to make use of it.

We'll come back to the question of hindsight shortly, but I want first to acknowledge another respect in which the argument of the book is incomplete, and I can now develop it a little further. I am not the first to claim that until fairly recently medicine did more harm than good: Shapin tells us that 'The Harvard biochemist L.J. Henderson [1878–1942] was supposed to have remarked "that it was only sometime between 1910 and 1912. . . that a random patient, with a random disease, consulting a doctor chosen at random, had, for the first time in the history of mankind, a better than 50–50 chance of profiting from the encounter."' Most historians of medicine have encountered this argument in some form, although for the most part they choose to ignore it: this is the price they must pay if they are to avoid writing about progress. The result is that there has been no serious debate about how much good traditional medicine did (if any), though Sheila Ryan Johansson has argued that medicine extended elite life expectancy in the period 1500 to 1800. I think she is mistaken: the improvements in life expectancy she attributes to medicine were, I would argue, attributable to improvements in diet and hygiene.

I am also not the first to claim that when pre-twentieth-century medicine worked it was by mobilizing the placebo effect. The claim was made by Arthur K. Shapiro and Elaine Shapiro in *The Powerful Placebo* (1997), and before them by W. R. Houston, writing in the *Annals of Internal Medicine* (1938). The Shapiro book is widely cited by doctors; it was reviewed in three medical history journals, but it has only once been cited in an article published in such a journal. Because they have avoided the question of how far traditional medicine worked, historians of medicine have also avoided the Shapiro thesis.

When I wrote *Bad Medicine* I did not for a moment imagine that the fact that Hippocratic medicine did more harm than good was *my* discovery. But I failed to say whose discovery it was. This was for the simple reason that I did not know. I was clear that Pierre-Charles-Alexandre Louis had not grasped that bloodletting necessarily did more harm than good. But who did first understand this simple fact? (It is, indeed, a fairly simple fact: it was apparent to Robert Boyle in the 1660s, although he was too frightened of the doctors to say so in print.) Standard histories of medicine do not address the question. The only clue I had when I wrote *Bad Medicine* was a passing reference by Carlo Cipolla to a Dr. Dietl in Vienna and a Dr. Bennett in Edinburgh. Now, belatedly, I can give them their place in my argument.

The classic English-language attack on bloodletting was written by John Hughes Bennett (1812–75), a professor at Edinburgh who is now remembered mainly for having given the first account of leukaemia as a blood disorder. 'Observations on the Results of an Advanced Diagnosis and Pathology applied to the Management of Internal Inflammations' appeared in the *Edinburgh Medical Journal* in 1857. Hughes Bennett was drawing on the work of Jospeh Dietl, *Der Aderlass in den Lungenentzundungen* or *Bloodletting in Pneumonia* (1849). Dietl and Hughes Bennett were the first to produce statistical evidence comparing treatment with bloodletting with no treatment, or with what amounted to placebo treatment, and to show that no treatment was markedly preferable to traditional treatment. (In 1851, in a work unavailable to Hughes Bennett, Dietl showed that bloodletting tripled the death rate in pneumonia).

Hughes Bennett ought to be an important figure in any history of medicine, for not only was his attack on bloodletting decisive (or at least it should have been—as we have seen, Osler was once again recommending bloodletting in pneumonia in 1892), but he was one of the first in Britain to place the microscope at the centre of a medical education. The date of his work on bloodletting is important: traditional therapy still retained an intellectual credibility until the middle of the nineteenth century, right up to the revolution represented by germ theory. Once the old fantasy technology had finally been abandoned, it took only a decade to produce a medicine that really worked. But Hughes Bennett, statistician and microscopist, had no part in that revolution. Dietl, having recognized the deleterious effects of traditional therapies, turned to hydrotherapy—at least he stopped doing harm. Hughes Bennett took a different path. He put his faith in the idea of a new medical science, but unfortunately he had an uncanny ability to make the wrong choices. In 1857 he was proselytizing for the chemistry of Justus von Liebig: this was two years after Snow had shown, in the case of cholera, that one had to think of infectious diseases as caused by organisms (or something similar), not, as the followers of von Liebig claimed, by poisons (or something similar). Hughes Bennett then turned to work on the Pasteur-Pouchet debate. He produced a learned and persuasive article ('The Atmospheric Germ Theory', *Edinburgh Medical Journal*, 13 [1868], 810–34), based on his own elaborate and painstaking experiments, an article proving that Pasteur was wrong and Pouchet was right. He published this ambitious article the year after Lister first published on antiseptic surgery, putting Pasteur's germ theory of putrefaction to work, and it seems improbable that Hughes Bennett had not already heard of the work Lister was doing in Glasgow, just a few miles away (though he cites only Lister's early article on the pigmentation of the skin of frogs).

Hughes Bennett is a striking example of how easy it is to back the wrong side during a scientific revolution. I recommend him to historians of medicine who want to write history without hindsight. Advocates of the symmetry principle may find it interesting to give an account of Hughes Bennett's contribution to the spontaneous generation debate written on the assumption that *he may have been right, and Lister may have been wrong*. It is perfectly possible to write such an account, providing we leave out a fact that we can only know through hindsight, now that the debate about spontaneous generation has finally been settled, a fact that was invisible to Hughes Bennett and is therefore missing from the historical record: Hughes Bennett's techniques for sterilizing his experimental equipment were inadequate. (Since he believed no living creature could survive a temperature of 100° C it is likely that he skimped on the procedures advocated by Pasteur.)

Hindsight is sometimes not just permissible but indispensable. You cannot write the *history* of a scientific dispute until you know the outcome, because until then the basic facts are in dispute. If you intervene in a scientific dispute before it is over, you are writing science, not history. If you were to write, after the outcome is known, pretending the facts might be other than they are—that the sun might go round the earth, or germs generate spontaneously—then you would be writing science fiction, not history. There *are* varieties of history that you can write without employing hindsight. History of science is not one of them.

If I were writing *Bad Medicine* now, Hughes Bennett would have a central place in my story. So would an obscure eighteenth-century doctor, William Taplin (1740?–1807). By 1789 Taplin was well on his way to making his fortune by marketing pills for horses: in that year his *Gentleman's Stable Directory* appeared in its ninth edition. But before he became a farrier, Taplin had evidently tried to make a living in medicine, and in 1789 he published under a pseudonym ('Gregory Glyster, an old practitioner') a humorous work, *The Æsculapian labyrinth explored; or, medical mystery illustrated* (retitled in its third edition *A Dose for the Doctors*). This wonderful little book should be read by every historian of medicine.

One of the central questions raised in *Bad Medicine* is how traditional medicine survived when it did no good. Half of the answer is provided by the mobilization of the placebo effect; but the other half of the answer is that doctors learnt to mislead their patients into thinking they were doing good when they were in fact doing harm, just as astrologers learnt to adapt their horoscopes to the hopes and fears of the individuals they had in front of them. I was clear when I wrote *Bad Medicine* that traditional medicine was an elaborate confidence trick, one which deceived doctors as well as patients. But where could one find an account of how the trick was performed? The answer is in Taplin's *Æsculapian Labyrinth*. The purpose of the book is to instruct every sort of medical practitioner (doctors, surgeons, men midwives, apothecaries) on how to maximize their income. Taplin writes on the assumption that actually curing patients is completely irrelevant to success: what matters is creating the right image. So a doctor should seem always to be in a hurry, and should keep a carriage standing at his door, so that prospective patients will be convinced that he is in constant demand. He should never return in his carriage by the same route as he drove out, for he needs to be seen on his rounds by as many people as possible. When visiting a patient you must

> take care to *look* wisdom in every feature; speak but little, and let it be impossible *that little* should be understood; let every hint, every *shrug* be carefully calculated to give the hearers a wonderful opinion of your learning and experience.—In your *half-heard* and mysterious conversation with your *medical inferior* [the apothecary], do not forget to drop a few observations upon—'the animal oeconomy'—'circulation of the blood'—'acrimony'—'the non naturals'—'stricture upon the parts'—'acute pain'—'inflammatory heat'—'nervous irritability', and all those *technical traps* that fascinate the hearers, and render the patient yours ad libitum.

The doctor must adapt himself to the rank of his patients, 'regulating your behaviour. . . from the *most* pompous *personal ostentation*, to the meanest and *most contemptible servility.*' If you are a surgeon you should display in your consulting room a profusion of skeletons and of anatomical specimens, 'both wet and dry'. 'Remember to let the *certificates* of your professional qualifications, from your different *lecturing tutors*, be so placed (in elegant frames) as to meet the eye in a conspicuous direction. . .'

 The Æsculapian Labyrinth is a satire, but Taplin chooses to abandon his pose of deepest cynicism at the end: 'A steady observance of the iniquity of medical practice has long since powerfully convinced me of the absolute necessity of professional reformation'; in the meantime his goal is to arm 'the public with a weapon of self-defence.' Of course his is not an unbiased, objective account of the practice of medicine in the eighteenth century—but it tells us more about the doctor–patient relationship in the centuries before antibiotics than any medical textbook. And it reminds us that the call for professional reformation is as old as the practice of medicine: there never was a time when everyone was taken in by the doctors.

The key obstacle to medical progress, this book has argued, was not economic self-interest, for, as Taplin recognized, new science was every bit as good as old for entrapping patients; nor was it some insuperable intellectual obstacle; it was the cultural identity of the medical profession, an identity transmitted through the texts of Hippocrates and Galen, and symbolized by the leech, the lancet, and the tourniquet. What held doctors captive was an imaginary world of their own creation, and the history of medicine may end as a history of science, but it needs to begin as a history of the medical imagination. The idea of such a history may seem a strange one, but it is an idea as old as the modern idea of science, and any attempt to distinguish between real sciences and fantasy sciences leads straight to it. In *Novum Organum* (1620), Francis Bacon described a number of ways in which the human mind can be led astray. He gives each of these sources of error the name of Idols because, like a believer worshipping a false god, we go astray while convinced we are still on the right road. The last source of error is what he calls the Idols of the Theatre:

> Lastly, there are Idols which have immigrated into men's minds from the various dogmas of philosophies, and also from wrong laws of demonstration. These I call Idols of the Theatre, because in my judgment all the received systems are but so many stage plays, representing worlds of their own creation after an unreal and scenic fashion.

★★★

FURTHER READING

I have organized this short guide to further reading according to the Parts into which the book is divided. Further bibliography, references, and links to other websites can be found at www.badmedicine.co.uk.

INTRODUCTION

The late Roy Porter is undoubtedly the most influential medical historian of the last few decades. See in particular his *The Greatest Benefit to Mankind: A Medical History of Humanity from Antiquity to the Present* (London, 1997). Another very useful standard history is Irvine Loudon (ed.), *Western Medicine: An Illustrated History* (Oxford, 1997). For a doctor's view of the history of medicine see Raymond Tallis, 'The Miracle of Scientific Medicine', in his *Hippocratic Oaths: Medicine and its Discontents* (London, 2004), 17–24. The key critique of modern medicine is Ivan Illich, *Limits to Medicine* (London, 1976). On the Oath, Howard Markel, " 'I Swear By Apollo' – On Taking the Hippocratic Oath," *New England Journal of Medicine*, 350 (2004), 2026–9.

I. THE HIPPOCRATIC TRADITION

The main primary sources are: *Hippocratic Writings*, ed. G. E. R. Lloyd (London, 1978); Galen, *Selected Works*, tr. P. N. Singer (Oxford, 1997); Charles Singer, *Galen, On Anatomical Procedures* (Oxford, 1956). Highly recommended is Jacques Jouanna, *Hippocrates* (Baltimore, 1999). Shigeshisa Kuriyama, *The Expressiveness of the Body and the Divergence of Greek and Chinese Medicine* (New York, 1999) is exceptionally thought-provoking.

For a survey of the Middle Ages, Nancy G. Siraisi, *Medieval and Early Renaissance Medicine* (Chicago, 1990). A wonderful book on pre-scientific medicine is Barbara Duden, *The Woman beneath the Skin: A Doctor's Patients in Eighteenth-Century Germany* (Cambridge Mass., 1991). To understand what doctors were really doing, read Daniel Moerman, *Meaning, Medicine and the 'Placebo Effect'* (Cambridge, 2002), or, more briefly, chapter 2 of Harry Collins and Trevor Pinch, *Dr Golem: How to Think about Medicine* (Chicago, 2005).

II. REVOLUTION POSTPONED

For a good general survey of the early modern period, see Roger French, *Medicine before Science: The Business of Medicine from the Middle Ages to the Enlightenment* (Cambridge, 2003). There are a number of helpful books on Renaissance advances in anatomy: Bernard Schultz, *Art and Anatomy in Renaissance Italy* (Ann Arbor, 1985); Andrew Cunningham, *The Anatomical Renaissance* (Aldershot, 1997); Andrea Carlino, *Books of the Body* (Chicago, 1999); R. K. French, *Dissection and Vivisection in the European Renaissance* (Aldershot, 1999). Also on vivisection, see Anita Guerini, 'The Ethics of Animal Experimentation in Seventeenth-Century England', *Journal of the History of Ideas*, 50 (1989), 391–407.

There is a fine digital replica of Vesalius's *Fabrica* available from www.octavo.com. The standard authority is C. D. O'Malley, *Andreas Vesalius of Brussels, 1514-1564* (Berkeley, Calif., 1964). A valuable article is Katharine Park, 'The Criminal and the Saintly Body: Autopsy and Dissection in Renaissance Italy', *Renaissance Quarterly*, 47 (1994), 1–33.

Harvey can be read in William Harvey, *The Circulation of the Blood and Other Writings* (London, 1963). An excellent short introduction to the extensive literature on Harvey is Andrew Gregory, *Harvey's Heart* (Cambridge, 2001). C. R. S. Harris, *The Heart and the Vascular System in Ancient Greek Medicine* (Oxford, 1973) puzzles over why the ancient Greeks (including Galen) did not discover the circulation of the blood.

On theories of contagion, see Carlo M. Cipolla, *Miasmas and Disease: Public Health and the Environment in the Pre-Industrial Age* (New Haven, 1992); Vivian Nutton, 'The Seeds of Disease: An Explanation of Contagion and Infection from the Greeks to the Renaissance', *Medical History*, 27 (1983), 1–34; Vivian Nutton, 'The Reception of Fracastoro's Theory of Contagion: The Seed that Fell among Thorns?', *Osiris*, 6 (1990), 196–234; and Lise Wilkinson, 'Rinderpest and Mainstream Infectious Disease Concepts in the Eighteenth Century', *Medical History*, 28 (1984), 129–50.

Three postscripts to my discussion of theories of animate contagion. 1) I am not the first to turn from Nardi to Platter (above, p. 128). The anonymous annnotator of the 1714 edition of Creech's translation of Lucretius (which advertises itself as 'a complete system of the Epicurean philosophy' and was reprinted in 1722) added (apparently as an afterthought) a note 'Of Contagion, the chief Cause of a Plague' (II, 776–81) in which he reports Platter's views with care. He stresses that Platter has an account of how 'resistance' to disease may vary, and that he argues that there may be asymptomatic carriers of diseases—in other words he fully recognizes what we would think of as distinctively 'modern' aspects of Platter's theory. 2) I was too quick to accept the Singers' account of theories of animate contagion after 1725 (above, p. 129). See the excellent article by M. E. De Lacy and A. J. Cain, 'A Linnean Thesis Concerning *Contagium Vivum*: the "Exanthemata viva" of John Nyander and its place in contemporary thought', *Medical History*, 39 (1995), 159–85 (discussing a text of 1757). Nyander and his contemporary Plenciz provoked William Alexander (who had published *Experimental Essays . . . on the External Application of Antiseptics* in 1768) to devise a series of experiments to refute the germ theory of putrefaction. See his *An Experimental Enquiry* (1771), ch. 8: 'Of Animalcula, Whether the Cause or the Effect of Putrefaction', pp. 87–155. See also Anon., *Necessary to All Families* (1788), which provides a full account of animate contagion. 3) In my discussion of Spallanzani (above p. 131) I suggested it was difficult to grasp that microscopic creatures could have macroscopic effects; but this very difficulty was soon to be discussed and overcome by James Tytler, in *A Treatise on the Plague and Yellow Fever* (1799), 188–9. These three postscripts deepen the puzzle as to why germ theory failed to win support before Pasteur and Lister.

On the microscope, Brian J. Ford, *The Leeuwenhoek Legacy* (Bristol, 1991) is fundamental, if hard to obtain. Catherine Wilson, *The Invisible World: Early Modern Philosophy and the Invention of the Microscope* (Princeton, 1995), is an excellent survey. Also useful is Edward G. Ruestow, *The Microscope in the Dutch Republic* (Cambridge, 1996).

The Conclusion draws especially on Andrew Wear, *Knowledge and Practice in English Medicine, 1550–1680* (Cambridge, 2000) and on Gianna Pomata, *Contracting a Cure: Patients, Healers and the Law in Early Modern Bologna* (Baltimore, 1998).

III. MODERN MEDICINE

James Le Fanu, *The Rise and Fall of Modern Medicine* (London, 1999) understands that modern medicine is fundamentally different from everything that preceded it. On the nineteenth century in general, W. F. Bynum, *Science and the Practice of Medicine in the Nineteenth Century* (Cambridge, 1994). On "first do no harm", Cedric M. Smith, "Origin and Uses of *Primum Non Nocere*", *Journal of Clinical Pharmacology*, 45 (2005), 371–8. On physiology and vivisection, Claude Bernard, *An Introduction to the Study of Experimental Medicine*, tr. Henry Copley Greene (New York, 1957); Michel Foucault, *The Birth of the Clinic* (London, 1973); John E. Lesch, *Science and Medicine in France: The Emergence of Experimental Physiology, 1790–1855*

(Cambridge, Mass., 1984); Richard D. French, *Anti-vivisection and Medical Science in Victorian Society* (Princeton, 1975); Stewart Richards, 'Anaesthetics, Ethics and Aesthetics: Vivisection in the Late Nineteenth-Century British Laboratory', in Andrew Cunningham and Perry Williams (eds.), *The Laboratory Revolution in Medicine* (Cambridge, 1992), 142–69.

On the birth of controlled trials and of medical statistics, the key sources are to be found at www.jameslindlibrary.org: a wonderful resource. See also Kenneth Carpenter, *History of Scurvy* (Cambridge, 1986); Stephen R. Bown, *Scurvy* (Chichester, 2003)—but see Nick Rodger, *The Wooden World* (London, 1986) and Glyn Williams, *The Prize of All the Oceans* (London, 1999) on deaths at sea; P. C. A. Louis, *Researches on the Effects of Bloodletting in Some Inflammatory Diseases* (Birmingham, Al., 1986); Andrea A. Rusnock, *Vital Accounts: Quantifying Health and Population in Eighteenth-Century England and France* (Cambridge, 2002). On trials comparing conventional medicine with homeopathy, see Michael Emmans Dean, *The Trials of Homeopathy* (Essen, 2004). A valuable collection of articles is Gérard Jorland *et al.* ed., *Body Counts: Medical Quantification in Historical and Sociological Perspectives* (Montreal, 2005): see, for example, the essay by Ulrich Tröhler. On the survival of bloodletting, Chantal Beauchamp, *Le sang et l'imaginaire médical: Histoire de la saignée aux XVIIIe et XIXe siècles* (Paris, 2000), and Guenter B. Risse, 'The Renaissance of Bloodletting: A Chapter in Modern Therapeutics,' *Journal of the History of Medicine*, 34 (1979), 3–22. On Haygarth, Christopher Booth, *John Haygarth FRS* (Philadelphia, 2005).

On spontaneous generation, John Farley, *The Spontaneous Generation Controversy from Descartes to Oparin* (Baltimore, 1974) is more narrowly focused than the title would suggest. On Needham, there is Shirley A. Roe, 'John Turberville Needham and the Generation of Living Organisms', *Isis*, 74 (1983), 159–84. Pasteur and Pouchet are dealt with briefly in chapter 4 of Harry Collins and Trevor Pinch, *The Golem: What Everyone Should Know about Science* (Cambridge, 1993). John Tyndall has been reprinted: *Essays on the Floating-Matter of the Air* (Delanco, NJ, 2003).

On germ theory, John Waller, *The Discovery of the Germ* (Cambridge, 2002) provides a quick survey. Margaret Pelling, *Cholera, Fever and English Medicine, 1825–1865* (Oxford, 1978) has been influential. In the same tradition, Michael Worboys, *Spreading Germs: Disease Theories and Medical Practice in Britain, 1865–1900* (Cambridge, 2000).

On Snow, Peter Vinten-Johansen, Howard Brody, Nigel Paneth, Stephen Rachman, Michael Rip, *Cholera, Chloroform and the Science of Medicine: A Life of John Snow* (Oxford, 2003), and (rather missing the point), Howard Brody, Michael Rip, Peter Vinten-Johansen, Nigel Paneth, Stephen

Rachman, 'Map-Making and Myth-Making in Broad Street: The London Cholera Epidemic, 1854', *Lancet*, 356 (2000), 64–8.

On childbed fever, Irvine Loudon, *The Tragedy of Childbed Fever* (Oxford, 2000), Oliver Wendell Holmes, *Medical Essays* (Boston, 1911), and Ignaz Semmelweis, *The Etiology, Concept, and Prophylaxis of Childbed Fever*, tr. K. Codell Carter (Madison, 1983).

On Pasteur, Gerald L. Geison, *The Private Science of Louis Pasteur* (Princeton, 1995) and Bruno Latour, *The Pasteurization of France* (Cambridge, Mass., 1988).

On Lister, Richard B. Fisher, *Joseph Lister, 1827–1912* (London, 1977).

On Fleming, Gwyn MacFarlane, *Alexander Fleming: The Man and the Myth* (Cambridge, Mass., 1984) and Wai Chen, 'The Laboratory as Business: Sir Almroth Wright's Vaccine Programme and the Construction of Penicillin', in Andrew Cunningham and Perry Williams (eds.), *The Laboratory Revolution in Medicine* (Cambridge, 1992), 245–92.

A useful book for thinking about methodological and theoretical issues is Stanley J. Tambiah, *Magic, Science, Religion and the Scope of Rationality* (Cambridge, 1990).

IV. AFTER CONTAGION

On lung cancer, *Unfiltered: Conflicts Over Tobacco Policy and Public Health*, ed. Erich A. Feldman and Ronald Bayer (Cambridge, Mass., 2004), and Charles Webster, 'Tobacco Smoking Addiction: A Challenge to the National Health Service', *British Journal of Addiction*, 79 (1984), 8–16.

For the McKeown thesis, Thomas McKeown, *The Modern Rise of Population* (London, 1976). There is a recent survey of the issues in James C. Riley, *Rising Life Expectancy: A Global History* (Cambridge, 2001). I have found the following particularly helpful for the nineteenth century: Henry Abelove, 'Some Speculations on the History of Sexual Intercourse during the Long Eighteenth Century in England', in his *Deep Gossip* (Minneapolis, 2003), 21–8; Georges Vigarello, *Concepts of Cleanliness: Changing Attitudes in France since the Middle Ages* (Cambridge, 1988); Simon Szreter, 'The Importance of Social Intervention in Britain's Mortality Decline c.1850–1914: A Re-interpretation of the Role of Public Health', *Social History of Medicine*, 1 (1988), 1–37, with reply by Sumit Guha, 'The Importance of Social Intervention in England's Mortality Decline: The Evidence Reviewed', *Social History of Medicine*, 7 (1994), 89–113; Robert W. Fogel, 'The Conquest of High Mortality and Hunger in Europe and America: Timing and Mechanisms', in Patrice Higonnet, David Landes, and Henry Rosovsky (eds.), *Favorites of Fortune* (Cambridge, Mass., 1991), 33–71. For the twentieth century, J. P. Bunker, 'Medicine Matters After All', *Journal of the Royal College of Physicians of London*, 29 (1995), 105–12, and Johan P. Mackenbach, 'The Contribution of Medical Care to Mortality Decline: McKeown Revisited', *Journal of Clinical Epidemiology*, 49 (1996), 1207–13.

POSTSCRIPT

On questions of method, Ian Hacking, *The Social Construction of What?* (Boston, 1999); my review of Paul Boghossian, *Fear of Knowledge* (Oxford, 2006) on www.socialaffairsunit.org; and my reply to Shapin, *London Review of Books*, 14 Dec. 2006. On Hughes Bennett, John Harley Warner, 'Therapeutic Explanation and the Edinburgh Bloodletting Controversy: Two Perspectives on the Medical Meaning of Science in the Mid-Nineteenth Century,' *Medical History* 24 (1980), 241–58 and L. S. Jacyna, ' "A Host of Experienced Micropscopists": the Establishment of Histology in Nineteenth Century Edinburgh,' *Bulletin of the History of Medicine* 75 (2001), 225–53. Eugeniusz Kucharz, 'The life and achivements of Joseph Dietl,' *Clio Medica* 16 (1981), 25–35. Michael Hunter, 'Boyle versus the Galenists,' *Medical History* 41 (1997), 322–61. Milton Wainwright and Harold T. Swan, 'C. G. Paine and the earliest surviving clinical records of penicillin therapy,' *Medical History* 30 (1986), 42–56. Sheila Ryan Johansson, *Death and the Doctors: Medicine and Elite Mortality in Britain from 1500 to 1800* (Cambridge, 1999). I owe my knowledge of Taplin to Michael MacKay.

INDEX

Note: Page numbers in *italics* indicate illustrations